2.50

SO-BUH-360

DRUGS & THE LAW:
the Canadian Scene

RICHARD A. BOGG

Division of Health Services Administration
Clinical Sciences Building
The University of Alberta
Edmonton 61, Alberta, Canada

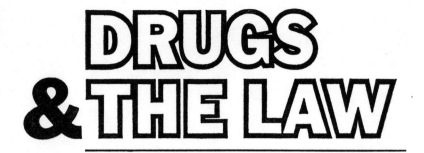

DRUGS & THE LAW

the Canadian Scene

REGINALD WHITAKER

METHUEN

TORONTO LONDON SYDNEY WELLINGTON

Copyright © 1969 by Methuen Publications
(A Division of the Carswell Company Limited)

All rights reserved. No part of this publication
may be reproduced, stored in a retrieval system
or transmitted in any form or by any means, electronic,
mechanical, photocopying, recording or otherwise,
without the prior written permission of
Methuen Publications, 145 Adelaide Street West,
Toronto, Canada.

Library of Congress Catalog Card Number 78-94434
SBN   458   90160/1   hc
SBN   458   90320/5   pb

Printed and bound in Canada
1   2   3   4   5   73   72   71   70   69

Contents

Preface

In an introduction to a book by an American philosopher concerning his experiences with LSD and other hallucinogenics, Dr. Timothy Leary advises the readers that unless they have taken LSD they will not understand what the author is saying. That statement clearly defines what this book is *not*. It is not a view from inside the drug subculture. The view is from the outside looking in; but it is, on the whole, a sympathetic view, although one not uncolored by criticism. It is less sympathetic to the law makers, for if drug abuse is dangerous and harmful to the individual, laws to combat drug abuse are just as often dangerous and harmful to the individual. Governments should know better.

Drug abuse is not an isolated phenomenon. If we have a drug problem it is not because a group of persons have, by becoming drug users, wilfully created a problem where none existed before. Competent medical doctors seek to separate the mere symptoms of a disease from its underlying causes. Only a quack would attempt to cure a brain tumour by prescribing aspirin. Yet just such quackery runs rampant in Parliament or in the provincial legislatures when a social problem such as drug addiction or drug abuse arises. The answer is always to suppress the immediate symptoms, to stop people sticking needles in their arms, inhaling marijuana, swallowing LSD, or sniffing glue. It is widely believed that an Act of Parliament is like a magic curse which, when laid upon the offending behavior, will cause it to vanish. "I can call spirits from the vasty deep," boasted Glendower. To which Hotspur quite rightly replied, "Why so can I, or so can any man. But will they come when you do call for them?"

Symptoms of a disease are unpleasant and upsetting. But they are also helpful warning signs that all is not well beneath the surface. Drug addiction, drug abuse, drug cults – all these are symptoms of deeper problems of our society. If we set all our energies merely to suppress these symptoms, or if we view the treatment of drug users as being the 'adjustment' of their personalities to conform to the majority, then we will ultimately defeat our own intentions, not to speak of damaging the hearts and minds of many people along the way. So long as drug use and drug users are treated as an isolated phenomenon, as a 'problem' which can be 'solved' by the application of some technical gimmickry, then it can be said with all certainty that no solution will be found. Nor will a solution ever be found until it is recognized that the problem does not begin with the individuals who happen to be the targets of law enforcement, that its roots run very much deeper, that the drug problem raises serious questions about a society in which all of us are implicated. When a chain-smoking, whisky-drinking, pill-swallowing judge sentences an eighteen year-old to spend a year in prison for being caught with a small quantity of marijuana, it is entirely legitimate to ask just what the hell is going on.

Parliament, the press, the public, are all very much concerned with the issue of drugs. A special committee has been set up by the Federal government to undertake a two-year study of the entire question. The information with which the average person is bombarded is conflicting, confusing, and ultimately baffling. Beyond this, there lies the fact that the use of drugs to create artificial paradises of the mind is an activity profoundly unsettling to our culture, as unsettling as sex and violence and revolution. What is needed is a broader perspective within which the political issue of drugs can be placed. This book is an attempt to draw such a perspective.

It is a commonplace that we live in an age of specialization. To achieve a perspective on the drug issue it is necessary to examine medical, biochemical, pharmacological, psychological, sociological, political, legal and philosophical evidence. It is legitimate to inquire as to the qualifications of someone attempting such a comprehensive inquiry who is not himself a doctor, biochemist, pharmacologist, psychologist, sociologist, lawyer or philosopher. But in fact the pharmacologists are apt to avoid saying anything about sociology; the lawyers shy away from biochemistry; the psychologists shun philosophy; the political scientists are quite indifferent to pharmacology. The result is that the story is told in bits and pieces, which appear in unrelated journals, and the ordinary interested person lacks the time or the dedication to hunt down all this information and to put it within a broader picture. In fact, as politics and government intrude more and more into the details of our daily lives – in this case into the question of which substances people should be allowed to consume and which they should not – it becomes less and less safe to 'leave it to the experts'. If this book provokes any of the experts to defend contrary viewpoints within a broader framework than is usual within any of their specialized fields, then all to the better.

While I have drawn on a wide variety of existing studies, I have not attempted a 'scientific' investigation into the drug scene in Canada today. Many impressions gathered from my own experiences and inquiries have been incorporated, but I would not raise these impressions to the dignity of scientific observations. For this reason I have refrained from indulging in the numbers game which so pleases the media, viz. – how many kids smoke pot; what percentage of students have taken LSD, etc. Anything short of a nation-wide inquiry with the full support of government and law enforcement agencies is unlikely to turn up an estimate of drug use which is anything but a guess. Until such an inquiry is undertaken, I think it better not to throw around too many loose figures – and so long as the drug use in question remains illegal, it is unlikely that *any* inquiry will be very accurate.

Finally, a personal note. I am not much of a drug-taker, either of the underground or the aboveground variety. I tend to be much happier in my normal state of consciousness than in an artificially created one. But I do not accept that this necessarily gives me, or anyone else, the right to declare that the behavior of those who think differently in this matter is obviously immoral and ought to be banned. All too often when people confront unfamiliar behavior, their reaction is that "there ought to be a law". Sometimes new laws may be necessary; but sometimes, perhaps, it would be better to have fewer laws.

Drugs and Society

1

The word *drug* conjures up ambivalent feelings in most people. We live in a highly drug-oriented society, where the idea is widely accepted that there is, or ought to be, a pill for every problem – aspirin for headaches, tranquillizers for anxiety, pep pills for depressions, sleeping pills for insomnia, and of course the final solution to overpopulation, known simply as The Pill. The pharmaceutical industry has become a major component of the economy, and the corner drug store is as common a sight as the corner confectionery. There is always some new 'wonder' drug being unveiled to combat some human affliction or other, real or imagined. School children are taught about the discoverers of the great drugs with the same reverence that in the Middle Ages was lavished on the Holy Fathers of the Church.

But at the same time, the word *drug* also has dark, disquieting connotations. *Drug addicts, the drug menace, teenage drug use, drugs on the campus, drug peddlars* – in headlines and in news broadcasts, these warnings surface like ugly and unwanted monsters from an unknown sea, and North American society – particularly middle-aged and middle-class North American society – is frightened. What does it all mean? Why are all these young people being arrested? Why can't we stop all this drug business?

Before any of these questions can be answered, it is first necessary to define our terms. *Drug* is by no means an easy word to define, and one could get into some very murky waters of pharmacology and biochemistry in the attempt. For our limited purposes we will settle for a loose definition of *drug* as a *chemical substance ingested by human beings that affects the working of the central nervous system*. This definition will by no means please specialists, for in some ways it is far too restrictive, and in others, far too lax. But it should suffice for the range of phenomena that this book sets out to examine. We are concerned only with drugs that alter the mind and thus alter human behavior – specifically drugs that are illegal or restricted under present Canadian legislation, but which seem to be in widespread use in defiance of the law.

A proper perspective on the whole problem can be very valuable. One wonders how many people who denounce teenage drug abuse over a friendly drink with an acquaintance realize that they themselves are consuming one of the most potent and dangerous mind-altering drugs known to man – a drug that in some parts of the world and in many eras of our own past has been denounced with as much moralistic venom as is vented on marijuana, LSD and even heroin today. How many people fully realize that the hearty beer or the elegent Pink Lady they hold in their hands is a substance that can cause mental derangement, physical degeneration, compulsive addiction, and death. Imagine for a moment that ethyl alcohol has just recently been discovered, that students and other such notorious groups are being reported as secretly using this drug. Inevitably the headlines would begin to appear: STUDENT DRINKS ALCOHOL: DRIVES CAR OFF BRIDGE; 15 YEAR OLD SEDUCED BY DRINK CRAZED GANG AT DRUNKEN ORGY; HIPPY BOOZE PEDDLAR ARRESTED: 12 BOTTLES SEIZED; DOCTOR SAYS ALCOHOL COULD CAUSE RED NOSE, LIVER DISEASES; COURT TOLD ALCOHOL-FIEND NEGLECTED WIFE, CHILD; AND TOUGH NEW LAWS PROMISED TO FIGHT RUM MENACE. In fact, most of the headlines would contain a kernel of truth. Alcohol *is* dangerous, and it is doubtful whether anyone can accurately estimate what the total social cost of alcoholism is, for the very reason that it is so extensive and pervasive. There are an estimated quarter million alcoholics in Canada, and one can only shudder at the amount of human suffering, let alone property damage, that could be traced to impaired driving. Yet Canadians annually spend more money on alcohol than they do on educating their children. A curious state of affairs and not a very solid moral base from which to criticize their children for self-indulgence.

On the other hand, young people who flaunt their pot smoking as a mark of superiority over their parents are seriously deluding themselves, if they believe that their habit is qualitatively different from getting drunk in the old-fashioned manner. For while the experience of inhaling marijuana does differ in detail from the experience of drinking alcohol, it is likely that the same basic motives underly the use of any drug to alter consciousness. And what is more, these motives run very deep, not only in our culture, but in almost all cultures, everywhere.

It is, as Aldous Huxley suggests, "strangely significant" that there are apparently no *naturally-occurring* narcotics, stimulants, or hallucinogenics whose properties were not discovered so long ago that a date can no longer be fixed to their origins. This would seem to suggest that the individual's dissatisfaction with mundane, everyday existence, with *reality* as we like to call it, is not limited to a few inadequate personalities, but is much more universal. People have always, and everywhere, prized any substance which offers a few moments escape from the imprisonment of the self, and from the tyranny of social convention. Even those who most moralistically oppose the evils of intoxication often provide a form of drug experience: the wild abandon of the revivalist meeting following a sermon against the Demon Rum.[1]

And yet such drugs, or drug-like experiences, are at the same time both necessary and dangerous. They provide a needed escape-valve for the pressures of social life, but also a temptation to the individual to drop out of social life altogether. Like sex, drugs are in the uneasy position of being both inside and outside the accepted social order: thus the inevitably ambivalent reaction of any society to these phenomena, and hence the elaborate rules and conventions set up to circumscribe and pacify the explosive potential inherent in them. As we live in an age of changing sexual practice, we are increasingly made aware of the artificial manner in which the sexual experience is controlled – monogamous marriage; taboos against pre-marital sex, adultery, incest, homosexuality; and perhaps most cunning of all, the manner in which children are brought up to regard sex as something so dangerous that it can only be handled in the socially sanctioned and defined fashion. It is on the latter point, however, that these elaborate arrangements have started to break down. For one reason or another fewer children of this generation seem to be accepting this viewpoint.

The case of drugs furnishes a close parallel to this changing attitude toward sex. One of the methods used by societies to manage the drug experience is to allow one or two drugs to assume an accepted place in social organization, elaborately bound about with ritual, religious significance, and strictly prescribed usage, and at the same time to violently oppose the use of any other unapproved drug. In this way, certain drugs have become assimilated into a culture, and thus pacified. The important point is that this process has very little to do with the pharmacology of the drug, but a great deal to do with the needs of the culture. Almost all known drugs, even those considered most dangerous to us, have an accepted place in some culture or other. And the reverse is also true. Hashish (or marijuana) has been accommodated in Middle Eastern Islamic society, while alcohol is a dreaded menace specifically proscribed by the Koran. Here in the West, of course, the exact opposite holds. Certain coca leaves were sacred to the ancient Incas, but cocaine, a derivative of coca, was once a dangerous drug among North American criminals. Indians of Western North America have elaborated an entire religious experience around the use of peyote, an LSD-like drug which we apparently feel to be extremely menacing, and yet the Indians are notoriously unable to handle alcohol.

In fact, the introduction of a new drug into a culture unprepared to cope with it can have a devastating effect. The settlers who took Canada from the Indians were well aware of this. The whisky bottle was a prime weapon in the campaign of cultural disorganization waged by the white invaders. On the other hand, cultural paranoia about strange drugs can also take on bizarre dimensions. Such an utterly innocuous substance as chocolate, for instance, roused a storm of violent disapproval when it was first introduced into Europe following its discovery in Mexico, on the absurd grounds that it was an aphrodisiac, and would lead its users, especially women, into a life of licence and debauchery.[2]

When coffee was first discovered in the Middle East, the official reaction was much the same as our present reaction to marijuana. In sixteenth century Egypt, sales were banned, stocks burned, persons were convicted of having drunk the evil substance, and warnings denouncing its pernicious properties were circulated widely. Eventually its use became so widespread that all the laws against it were repealed and coffee became a normal part of Middle Eastern life.[3] The use of tobacco in North America demonstrates even more vividly the cyclical nature of social responses to drugs. In the nineteenth century, a long struggle was waged against cigarettes, which led the *New York Times* to solemnly warn its readers in 1884 that "the decadence of Spain began when the Spaniards adopted cigarettes and if this pernicious practice obtains among adult Americans the ruin of the Republic is close at hand."[4] Gradually cigarette smoking has become so popular that strong social pressures are exerted to encourage people to smoke. Now that the connection between cigarettes and lung cancer has become apparent, the government is faced with the gargantuan task of trying to change the social mores so as to make smoking once again unpopular.

In a sense, certain drugs may take on symbolic meanings, as representing different styles of life. Alcohol in our society has delicate nuances of class designation attached to the various forms in which it is consumed: the beer-drinking worker in the pub is socially distant from the wine-tasting gourmet in the restaurant, and each is apt to have a low opinion of the other's tastes. Although both tea and coffee contain caffeine, tea is extremely popular in Britain, while coffee is virtually unchallenged in the United States (Canada, as always, rests somewhere between these two poles). Somehow the coffee break has become a characteristic of the North American work day, while 3 o'clock tea has remained specifically British. Cigars are associated with aggressive businessmen, and pipes, which were once considered a lower-class symbol, are now associated with the affluent college-educated elite.

Such symbolism, mild and imprecise enough when the drugs concerned are more or less approved, becomes much more formidable when the drug is one banned by the society. To the average North American, alcohol is the mark of the outgoing, aggressive, success-oriented personality so prized by business organizations. Conversely, the opium-smoking Oriental might seem to be a shiftless, lazy, good-for-nothing degenerate. To the Oriental, however, the smoking of opium might appear to impart a certain philosophical tranquillity, a passive dignity more in keeping with the traditional virtues than the crude, belligerent drunkenness of the North American.

The cultural relativism of any statements about drugs should now be clear. One would have to be either very ethnocentric or very foolhardy to make resoundingly absolute statements about any drugs based solely on one cultural perspective (and if we are honest with ourselves, one class or status position within that culture). Nor is it good enough to try to wriggle out of this dilemma by saying that whatever *our* culture says must at any rate be accepted for *us*, since the whole wrangle about drugs today turns precisely on the question of *what* our culture actually does say, and, perhaps more importantly who speaks for 'our culture' in the first place. This tangled knot must be faced up to later, but for now the reader may rest content in the knowledge that the queasy feeling he or she may be experiencing, of being entirely at sea, is one which most honest and open-minded investigators probably share. The problem is simply to keep afloat at an even keel, without sacrificing oneself either to complete relativism or to blind dogmatism.

The problem of *addiction* provides one example of the difficult course through which an investigator must pick his way. It might be thought that drugs could be divided into those which are addictive and those which are not. Unfortunately this type of distinction begins to dissolve when a detailed examination is made of the psychological processes involved in drug use. It is true that some drugs, such as heroin, cause physical changes in the body of the user which lead to withdrawal symptoms if administration of the drug ceases. It is also true that other drugs, such as marijuana, do not bring about such effects. But this by no means allows us to set up a rigid dichotomy of addictive/non-addictive drugs. Some people apparently use heroin without developing true physical dependence, while there are some people so habituated to using marijuana that its withdrawal will have serious consequences. Amphetamine users tend to exhibit certain signs of physical addiction, but these symptoms are so different from the typical symptoms of heroin addiction that the traditional definition of addiction must be considerably stretched.

In the face of these and similar ambiguities, the Expert Committee on Addiction-producing Drugs of the World Health Organization decided in 1964 to drop the distinction between *addiction* (physical) and *habituation* (psychological) in favour of a single term, *drug dependency* with the drug type specified. Drug dependency has been defined as a "state arising from repeated administration of a drug on a periodic or continuous basis. Its characteristics will vary with the agent involved and this must be made clear by designating the particular type of drug dependence in each specific case . . . ."[5] This is a much more flexible, and undoubtedly realistic, framework for the study of drug abuse. It is not without certain dangers, however, despite the Committee's own careful stipulation that the term "carries no connotation of the degree of risk to public health or need for a particular type of drug control." The danger arises not from the medical dimension of the definition, but from the unfortunate intermingling of medical and legal categories which plagues all attempts to illuminate this field. The law must, by its very nature, deal not with specific individuals, but with specific drugs. Any definition, such as the World Health Organization's, which tends to blur the distinction between say, heroin, marijuana, and alcohol provides a specious rationale both for those who would argue that marijuana use should be punished in exactly the same way as heroin use and for those who would argue that marijuana dependency is really no different from, say, dependency on an evening Martini. The skilled observer, of course, can readily distinguish between the person who drinks in a temperate fashion and one who develops into an alcoholic; between the person who smokes pot at an occasional party and one whose life is entirely centred around the marijuana experience; between someone who sniffs heroin with friends now and again and one who becomes completely addicted. All the law can do, however, is to categorize the drugs – heroin and marijuana are completely banned, alcohol is sold more or less freely to adults. As a result, 'A' may become a compulsive drinker, become ineffective in his job, ruin his health, make his home unbearable to wife and children, and perhaps end up being a burden on tax-supported health services, and at all times be perfectly within the law. Meanwhile, 'B', who mildly enjoys marijuana but feels no strong attraction, accepts a joint at a college party. The party is raided, 'B' is arrested, tried, convicted of being in possession of narcotics, and jailed.

The problem is not only that altogether too much emphasis has been put on the drugs and too little on the person, but that the law by nature is a very clumsy instrument to deal with such a complex phenomenon as drug dependency. In fact it might as well be made clear at this stage that any possible legal response to this problem will, by definition, be untidy and inconsistent. The conscientious legislator must divide up the drugs into various categories, and will hopefully do so with a view to the greatest social good. The conscientious doctor must deal with the individual problems of the individual persons, and since individuals differ, sometimes in the most extreme fashion, in their response to various drugs, the gap between the legal and the medical viewpoints will be both wide and inevitable.

There was once, so it is said, a happy age when governments defended the country from invasion, collected the garbage, cleared away the snow, delivered the mail, and otherwise minded their own business. Whether such an age really existed is open to question, but the drug issue would seem to indicate that the more government insinuates itself into the minute details of everyday life, the more untidy and less consistent its actions inevitably become. The old proverb had it best: "one man's meat is another man's poison." All that governments can do is to declare *this* substance officially "meat" and *this* officially "poison", and let the individuals take the consequences.

At this point the reader might suggest that surely a drug has certain specific pharmacological properties which will cause certain specific effects when taken. If you swallow a quantity of cyanide, your chances of living to tell about it are pretty close to nil. But the assumption of predictability of effects is not well justified with regard to the type of drugs with which we are concerned. What the drug user is seeking is a particular drug *experience*, and here the individual psychology of the user, and the entire set of cultural standards which the individual brings to bear in interpreting the physical effects of the drug would seem to be as important as the pharmacology of the drug itself. Those who have studied drug experiences tend to describe a threefold interaction between the drug, the expectations of the person taking the drug, and the environment in which it is taken. The question then becomes one of relative weight – which of these conditions is the most, and which the least, important. I am inclined to put more emphasis on the latter two conditions – the cultural and social aspects. Others may put more on the chemistry of the drug. This is a matter of legitimate dispute, and much more research is obviously needed before the matter can be settled.

It is important to recognize, however, that a certain moral judgment is implicit in either choice. Those who emphasize the drug are also apt to emphasize the frailty of human nature, and the necessity for a strong outside discipline to be exercised over the individual. Those who, like myself, emphasize the individual and his culture, tend to assume that a good deal of responsibility for personal freedom can be entrusted to the individual. It is most unfashionable now among social scientists to admit that moral judgments form the foundation of their theories, but the question of drugs is essentially and above all a moral issue, to be settled in the political arena on the basis of what is considered *right* and what is considered *wrong*. This book attempts to clear away some of the misrepresented 'facts', to bring forward some of the valid findings of medical and scientific studies, to point out some of the more obvious hypocrisies of contemporary laws and official attitudes, and to suggest the possibility of an alternative, and hopefully more sane, approach to the question of drug use. Ultimately, however, the moral decision must remain with the reader. In making this decision, however, the reader would do well to bear in mind the following warning from the U.S. Presidential Commission on Law Enforcement:

Mind-altering drug use is common to mankind. Such drugs have been employed for millennia in almost all cultures . . . we have been able to identify only a few societies in the world today where no mind-altering drugs are used; these are small and isolated cultures. Our own society puts great stress on mind-altering drugs as desirable products which are used in many acceptable ways. . . . In terms of drug use the rarest or most abnormal form of behavior is not to take any mind-altering drugs at all.[6]

Footnotes

[1]Aldous Huxley, *The Devils of Loudon: A Study in the Psychology of Power Politics and Mystical Religion in the France of Cardinal Richelieu* (New York, Harper and Row, 1952), pp. 313-15.

[2]Norman Taylor, *Narcotics: Nature's Dangerous Gifts* (New York, Dell, 1963), pp. 181-89.

[3]Robert S. DeRopp, *Drugs and the Mind* (New York, Grove Press, 1957), p. 248.

[4]Taylor, *op. cit.*, p. 104.

[5]World Health Organization, *Technical Report Series 273*, (1964).

[6]Richard H. Blum, "Mind-altering Drugs and Dangerous Behavior: Dangerous Drugs," in The President's Commission on Law Enforcement and Administration of Justice, *Task Force Report: Narcotics and Drug Abuse*, (Washington, D.C., United States Government Printing Office, 1967), p. 23.

Opiates: The Waters of Oblivion

2

"It is curious to reflect," suggests a British writer, "that many of our great-grandparents were junkies. In sickness or in depression, so letters and diaries of the last century tell us, the kindly family doctor prescribed opium and laudanum, or the parlour-maid was simply sent round the corner to the obliging chemist."[1] It is curious indeed when one considers that *dope fiends* have now sunk to a level of public ill repute somewhere below *sex perverts* and perhaps slightly above *Communists*. In fact most people, if pressed, would no doubt assert that narcotic addiction is some contemporary perversion, an unfortunate by-product of twentieth century progress, like air pollution or juvenile delinquency. In fact the problem is not so very new at all, and in many ways our sturdy forefathers, to whom we are always inclined to compare ourselves unfavorably in these matters, demonstrated at least an equal tendency to self-indulgence. It is an instructive exercise to examine the place of narcotics in nineteenth century life, as a means of putting the contemporary scene into perspective. Both the psychedelic cultists and the crusaders against the dope menace seem to be united on the assumption that the whole drug affair is something radically new and hitherto unheard of. In fact even the most superficial glance at its history discloses that, while there may be the odd new thing under the sun, novelty is, in truth, more apparent than real.

The opium poppy has been known to mankind for thousands of years. Exactly where its use first became known can no longer be determined. But the Greeks and the Romans were well aware of its pain-killing properties. A drug called *nepenthe*, probably an opiate, was described by Homer as a powerful destroyer of misery. The Latin name for the god of sleep was Morpheus (from which we derive the word *morphine*), who lived in a sunless land of silence, by the still waters of oblivion, round which poppies bloomed.[2] The young goddess Persephone was picking the blood-red flowers of the poppy plant when she was abducted by Hades, the god of death, and was from that time on condemned to spend three months of each year in the death-like sleep of the Underworld and nine months among the living on the earth.[3] That the allegory implied in this myth was widely understood can be seen in the warnings given by various learned Greeks against the addictive and destructive effects of the opium poppy.[4]

Public attitudes in the western world toward opium at the beginning of the nineteenth century were relatively uncommitted. But the drug gained in notoriety as addiction became more and more common among ordinary citizens, and particularly as it became associated with exotic and forbidden pleasures. It is the latter point that is particularly interesting, for it has parallels in contemporary drug problems. To those who may think that the paraphernalia of psychedelia flaunted by today's LSD cultists represents some shocking new aberration, it is interesting to note that opium attracted a somewhat similar cult among artists and intellectuals in the last century, with some of the same rationales that we hear today. Thomas de Quincey, whose *Confessions of an English Opium-Eater* was the first major piece of confessional literature from a drug addict, told how in 1804 he went to a druggist to relieve severe pains from which he was suffering and received a small package of opium. As a present-day hippy might say: it blew his mind.

Here was a panacea . . . for all human woes; here was the secret of happiness, about which philosophers had disputed for many ages, at once discovered; happiness might now be bought for a penny, and carried in the waistcoat-pocket; portable ecstasies might be had corked up in a pint-bottle; and peace of mind could be sent down by the mail.[5]

De Quincey, it should be pointed out, obviously shared one attitude with today's cultists; not only was opium good for *him* but it was immediately seen as a "panacea" for "*all* human woes". And what was more, cheap, bottled, instant salvation could, and should, be distributed to everyone. The LSD enthusiasts who talked excitedly a few years ago about dispensing their cure-all from bubble-gum machines were thus only introducing a new product, but not a new marketing concept.

Ten years after his first ecstatic experience, de Quincey had become thoroughly, and hopelessly, addicted.

From this date the reader is to consider me as a regular and confirmed opium-eater, of whom to ask whether on any particular day he had or had not taken opium would be to ask whether his lungs had performed respiration, or the heart fulfilled its functions.[6]

The exotic pleasures and imaginative delights that he at first secured from opium, so extravagantly detailed in his *Confessions*, soon turned to the most grisly nightmares. His attempts to free himself from the habit, were reported with scientific detail; but despite his claims to have triumphed, the evidence indicates that he continued using opium up to the very end of his life.[7] De Quincey's *Confessions*, couched as they were in rather sensationalist form, did much to create the image of the fanatical drug fiend, and his accounts of the heaven and hell to be found within a penny bottle must have imparted an aura of dread fascination to opium. Unfortunately, while subsequent scientific investigation has made his account of the 'ecstasies' of opium seem very dubious indeed, de Quincey has survived as a leading authority on the drug ever since.

Opium use was surprisingly widespread among nineteenth century writers. Edgar Allan Poe, Baudelaire, Keats, Wilkie Collins, Francis Thompson, and the poet Crabbe all used it regularly. Elizabeth Barrett Browning, Charles Dickens, and the composer Berlioz were some more prominent occasional users. After de Quincey, perhaps the best known opium addict was Coleridge, whose poem *Kubla Khan* has often been attributed to an ecstatic drug-induced dream. While it seems a senseless fallacy to attribute the poem to opium itself, as if the latter were a conscious entity, exactly this indeed happened, with a consequent enhancement of the alleged powers of the drug.

And all should cry, Beware! Beware!
His flashing eyes, his floating hair!
Weave a circle round him thrice,
And close your eyes with holy dread,
For he on honey-dew hath fed,
And drunk the milk of Paradise.[8]

At first Coleridge spoke of opium as "a spot of enchantment, a green spot of fountains and flowers and trees in the very heart of a waste of sands."[9] But later, like de Quincey, he became aware of its hellish side, and confessed bitterly that

I have in this one dirty business of Laudanum a hundred times deceived, tricked, nay, actually and consciously *lied*. And yet *all* these vices are so opposite to my nature, that but for this *Free-agency-annihilating* Poison, I verily believe that I should have suffered myself to have been cut to pieces rather than have committed one of them.[10]

There seems to have been a pattern to the visions that the Victorian writers experienced under opium. One image recurred again and again – an architectural vision of a cathedral or place or city, magnificent and alluring at first but soon turning into a menacing prison, where staircases end in mid-air or go on to ever more remote chambers, leading the frightened prisoner further and further inward, but never out.[11] Most artists, particularly those who had experienced the more romantic ecstasies, later turned savagely against opium as a hideous enslavement, but always with lingering nostalgia for the rapture of their early love.

It is a perplexing fact in the light of present-day medical knowledge of opiate reactions, that such hallucinatory visions and poetic torments should have been associated with a drug whose main pharmacological effect tends more toward the negative state of pain relief and the reduction of anxiety, rather than any positive kind of euphoria. Perhaps the secret of its appeal to the artistic mind lay in its power to reduce the individual to a half-waking state of twilight reverie where the mind's threshold of sensory awareness is lowered and dream-like thoughts mingle with reality. In this sense opium might have helped to facilitate the imaginative mechanisms of artistic creation, but it also ended by enslaving the persons who thought they were using it for their own ends. The view of opium as a magical elixir of imagination has not disappeared entirely, for the twentieth century French writer Jean Cocteau had described much the same relationship with opium as de Quincey experienced,[12] but for the most part the milk of paradise of *Kubla Khan* remains an historical curiosity, a monument to the extent to which a drug's effects may be created by the user's expectations. In the more mundane and prosaic twentieth century, most addicts refer straightforwardly to their drug as *junk* – as unromantic and unenchanting a name as could be imagined, but one perhaps more in keeping with the substance's real properties.

Despite its reputation as an essentially oriental vice, opium use was surprisingly widespread in both England and in North America in the nineteenth century. Medical science had not generally progressed to the point where the underlying disease mechanisms of afflicted persons could be isolated and dealt with. Consequently doctors were more often content to relieve the obvious symptoms causing discomfort. To this end opium was a true miracle drug, for whatever else one can say about it, it clearly does relieve pain. Unfortunately its addictive qualities were not so widely known; thus patent medicines were more often than not liberally laced with opiates, and children were often given opiates such as paregoric in the same way as children today are given cod-liver oil. By the 1890s, estimates of the number of addicted persons in the United States alone range from 400,000 to 1,500,000 or four per cent of the population.[13] By this time the dangers of opiate use were becoming recognized. Institutions sprang up around the turn of the century to meet the demand of addicts for cures. A typical issue of a North American magazine of this time might contain at least a half dozen advertisements for 'home cures' for addiction to opium, morphine, laudanum and other drugs. The significant point here is that at this time no terrible stigma was attached to addiction; 'cures' for addiction were offered alongside similarly dubious cures for alcoholism, asthma, rheumatism and baldness. In other words addiction was not at that time associated with criminality. An addict might come from any social level, including the most affluent, and addiction in itself did not necessarily lessen anyone's social respectability any more than did other unfortunate private vices such as alcoholism. So long as addicts received a sufficient amount of their drug, they continued as functioning members of society.

A disastrous by-product of the search for cures was the synthesis of heroin in 1898. Since morphine withdrawal symptoms were relieved by heroin, doctors at first believed it to be a cure for addiction. Inexplicably, it was not until 1910 that heroin's own potent addictiveness was understood. In the meantime the new drug had achieved wide distribution. This dismal failure of medical science must have done little to create confidence in the ability of medicine to deal with the addiction problem.

What then is this drug that has caused such human problems? Opium is a gummy black mixture drawn from the unripened seed capsules of the opium poppy by a most laborious and painstaking process. Opium contains numerous alkaloids, of which morphine and codeine are among the more potent. Heroin is an entirely synthetic drug, manufactured from morphine. *Opiates* is a term applied to all constituents of opium and may, for our purposes, be a somewhat more precise term than *narcotics* which, as a legal category under present-day law includes marijuana and cocaine which are not related pharmacologically to the opiates. Some, although not all, opiates have pain-killing properties and are potentially addictive.

Despite the lyricism of a de Quincey, a Coleridge, or a Cocteau, and despite the widespread prevalence of addiction in the late nineteenth century, it is nevertheless untrue that opiates are inherently attractive to everyone, and therefore represent a endemic danger to society. Research at Harvard indicated that the response of some ninety per cent of a normal population to an injection of morphine is not euphoria, but dysphoria (unpleasantness), with dizziness, nausea, itchiness, headache, mental clouding, and general unwelcome inertia as the main symptoms. Similar results were obtained with heroin.[14] In another experiment, 150 young non-addicts were given morphine doses; only three would voluntarily allow another dose, and none showed any positive interest in the drug. The researchers concluded that "opiates are not inherently attractive, euphoric or stimulant substances. The danger of addiction to opiates resides in the person, not in the drug."[15]

Where pain is already present, however, opiates can be extremely effective in bringing about relief – which is the basic reason for the widespread therapeutic use of morphine. When the drug is administered, a depression of the central nervous system results. There is some evidence that morphine is much less important for raising the actual pain threshold (the degree of pain stimulus necessary to cause a response) than it is for altering the reaction to pain. This is to say that pain is still perceived, but the mind's interpretation of the pain is changed because anxiety and alarm reactions are reduced. This hypothesis would seem to be confirmed by experiments in which patients already accustomed to morphine effects were given injections of a harmless salt solution which they were told was morphine, and proceeded to exhibit the same apparent relief from pain as demonstrated under morphine itself.[16] In other words, the pain-killing effects of opiates may be more psychological than physiological.

The exact process whereby an individual becomes addicted to

opiates remains to this day a matter of considerable controversy. It is a reflection of the political sensitivity of narcotics research, and of the ever present mythology surrounding the whole question, that so few substantive conclusions have been generally accepted to explain the phenomenon of addiction. Worse, there appears to be in much of the literature a venom toward opponents which exceeds even the usual formalized blood-letting of academic disputes. Those who defend established views tend to view critics as misguided fools or dangerous subversives, while dissenters are sometimes apt to characterize more orthodox authorities as mere apologists for repression. In short, 'scientific research' has by no means been untouched by the emotion-charged atmosphere which prevails in society as a whole when the question of narcotics is raised.

We may focus on certain symptoms of addiction about which most authorities are in agreement. It is clear that continuous injection of opiates results in the phenomenon of *tolerance*, which is a state of increased bodily resistance to the actions of the drug. Thus an experienced addict will require a dosage which would have been toxic in the early stages of his addiction in order to achieve the same desired effects. A second common factor is the appearance of *withdrawal symptoms*, which always appear when the addicted individual is unable to continue his injections. *Physical dependence* has been defined as "the development of an altered physiological state which requires continued administration of a drug to prevent the appearance of a characteristic illness, termed an 'abstinence syndrome' "[17] (of which withdrawal symptoms are part). *Psychological dependence* may be seen as a substitution of drug use for other forms of adaptive behavior. The drug becomes the solution to all problems.

Tolerance and withdrawal symptoms would seem to have a definitely physiological basis. Many persons have become addicted accidentally through medical treatment; moreover, animals have become addicted experimentally. Rats forced to drink a bitter morphine solution soon learned to choose the morphine over clear water and displayed definite signs of withdrawal illness when the morphine was removed. After a few weeks of withdrawal they even relapsed into morphine use when given the choice.[18] Other experiments have shown that rats will become addicted to morphine through self-injection when such an action is made possible.[19]

The withdrawal symptoms themselves are the most spectacular and distressing part of drug addiction. Many physicians and other observers have found it almost as shattering to watch as the addict must find the experience itself. Dr. Charles Terry, a pioneer in the study of addiction, told how in 1915, when the first strong anti-narcotics laws were passed in the United States, he watched the attempts of some sixty-five to seventy-five people to cure themselves in a hospital setting.

This is one of the experiences in my attempts to work out this problem which I do not like to recall . . . . We felt, as do most when contemplating drug addiction treatment, that a certain amount of suffering was necessary, but I was not prepared for the extreme suffering that I witnessed in these cases, nor was I prepared for one death which occurred in an apparently healthy woman. With the exception of two or three, all of these cases relapsed within a very short time after their discharge as cured, and I realized more than ever that here was indeed a medical problem and I began to harbor my first doubts as to the wisdom of blind restrictive legislation.[20]

There is a general pattern to withdrawal. From eight to twelve hours after the last dose, the addict becomes weak and restless and watery discharges come from the eyes and nose. There is shivering and sweating, and yawns that may become so violent that the jaw is dislocated. Cold goose flesh breaks out and stomach muscle contractions become so violent that they can be seen from the outside. Ferocious, blood-stained vomiting and constant diarrhoea continue for hours on end. A day and a half or so after the last dose the addict reaches his personal nadir. Racked by spasms and twitches, exhausted by lack of sleep, enfeebled and emaciated, wallowing in his own vomit, defecations, and mucous-like discharges, sometimes suffering constant involuntary orgasms, and possessed by a relentless and all-encompassing craving for his drug, the addict is a chilling sight. If he perseveres, he may begin making improvements within a week or so. At any time in this hellish process a single dose of morphine or heroin will render what appears to be a miraculous change in a matter of minutes: a subhuman example of extreme physical degeneration will suddenly become a perfectly normal and healthy individual.[21] A former middleweight boxing champion, Barney Ross, has described his withdrawal from morphine.

I saw elephants with horns on their heads. I saw animals jumping off cliffs. I saw mountains caving in and I saw rivers washing over big cities and drowning them. I saw rattlesnakes spitting out streams of poison.

I was covered with mud and I was being pushed down under the slime . . .
I couldn't breathe, the mud was in my mouth, it was going into my lungs
. . . I was choking . . . I screamed, "stop it, stop it!" In a fit of madness
I ran across the room and smashed my head into the wall.[23]

Addicts themselves usually speak of withdrawal, especially the 'cold
turkey' type just described, as an unimaginable misery. But there
are some doctors who are not impressed. Dr. Harris Isbell, who was
for years the Director of the Addiction Research Center located at
the Lexington, Kentucky treatment hospital for addicts, has stated
flatly that "whatever method of withdrawal is used, addicts will
complain," but that the withdrawal illness is a "self-limited condition
which, in individuals without organic disease, is never fatal".[23] Dr.
David Ausubel, who was also on the Lexington staff, has asserted
that although withdrawal symptoms are "undoubtedly uncomfortable" they are rarely worse than those of a "bad case of gastrointestinal influenza".[24] A bad case of 'flu', however, can sometimes
make an individual desperately ill. Perhaps a certain amount of
callousness is necessary in dealing with people as generally weak-
willed as drug addicts, but the addicts' own accounts of the experience should be listened to, and they are invariably terrifying.

At this point the reader might well be wondering why anyone
would want to put themselves in such a dangerous and distasteful
position. Unfortunately there is even less agreement about why
people begin using opiates than there is about the concept of addiction itself. The controversy seems to turn on the question of whether
positive euphoria or merely the negative avoidance of withdrawal
symptoms is what the addict seeks in continued use of opiates. The
popular conception, fostered by press reports of 'hopped-up dope
fiends' would seem to assume that opiate users experience compelling and forbidden pleasures from their drug. Certainly the writings
of de Quincey and Coleridge helped to shape this attitude. Moreover, the euphoria theory is not without its serious proponents
among psychologists and doctors. Dr. Ausubel, for instance, bases
his entire theory of addiction on the search for euphoria.[25] But since,
as already pointed out, opiates are not inherently attractive to most
people, then the taste for such euphoria must be of very limited
distribution in the general population. The psychological effects of
opiates in reducing unpleasant pain reactions would seem to be at
the root of their appeal to the small number of persons who seek
out their effects. To most people mere relief from pain is not an

experience fervently sought after except in unusual situations of illness or injury. But to some, the psychological processes set off by opiate ingestion would seem to be very effective in the reduction of all anxieties and tensions. In this sense, opiate 'euphoria' is a situation consciously desired but rather negative in its rewards. One of the most detailed studies of juvenile drug addiction undertaken, in New York city, concluded on this point that the opiate experience represents not a satisfaction but an elimination of desire.

De Quincey and others to the contrary notwithstanding, it is not an enjoyment of anything positive at all, and that it should be thought of as a 'high' stands as mute testimony to the utter destitution of the life of the addict with respect to the achievement of positive pleasures and of its repletion with frustration and unresolvable tension. It is in the main, an enjoyment of a nirvana-like state unprecedented and unenriched by the pleasure of getting there. It is an enjoyment of negatives . . . . Here, in 'the junkie paradise', they experience what Wikler has described as a diminution of their 'primary drives' of hunger, thirst, awareness of pain, and sexual tension. Their bodies are satisfied and sated.[26]

All this is important inasmuch as our present narcotics laws seem to be founded on the principle that addicts are extremely dangerous people whose very existence at large imperils the security of law-abiding citizens. The drives of 'normal' people may in this sense be far more dangerous. The sexual drive, for instance, may in some cases become so compelling that rape or other forms of sexual assault may result. But by analogy, what the addict seeks is not orgasm at all, but merely the subsequent state in which the sexual drive, with its attendant tensions, has been at least temporarily eliminated. The essentially harmless nature of people in such a state should be obvious. Nevertheless, the myth of the addict grasping for fiendish pleasures is unfortunately widespread, and underlies much public hysteria about drug addiction.

Whatever can be said of the positive rewards granted by the opiates to the novice user, once the mechanisms of addiction are set in motion, a new motive comes to the forefront – the brutal necessity to take more doses merely to avoid the recurring symptoms of withdrawal. One addict has stated that when she was *not* hooked, heroin made everything seem "all right", with worries all forgotten; but later, "all you're trying to do is keep from getting ill, really".[27] The reasons which attract an individual to opiates may in this sense be quite different from those which maintain and consolidate addiction.

One theory, advanced by Alfred Lindesmith of Indiana University, holds that the entire addiction process is based on the conscious use of opiates to relieve the physical distress of withdrawal symptoms. To be addicted in this sense means that the individual must be aware that the withdrawal symptoms will be alleviated by further use of the drug. In other words, an individual could develop withdrawal symptoms following opiate administration but would not be 'addicted' if he failed to connect his distress to the absence of the drug. Lindesmith thus tries to balance the physiological and psychological aspects of opiate use within one explanation. Moreover, he maintains that his theory explains addiction in universal terms, that it applies equally to a Chinese opium smoker and a North American junkie. The reasons which compelled de Quincey to eat opium are no doubt a world apart from the reason why an unemployed Vancouver slum-dweller starts shooting heroin – but in Lindesmith's theory, the cause of *addiction* itself remains exactly the same. Thus the euphoria experienced by addicts at the beginning of opiate use is, in Lindesmith's words, merely the "bait on the hook", the "hook" itself being the necessity of avoiding the agonies of withdrawal.[28] Unfortunately this theory cannot be used to predict what type of person is likely to become addicted.

It is important to realize that the physiological basis of addiction is only one part of any explanation of opiate use. One of the most startling findings of Dr. Chein and his associates in their detailed study[29] of addiction among New York delinquents was that of the eighty current heroin users that they studied, less than half were using the drug on a regular basis. In other words, a history of drug use and a psychological dependency on heroin were not always synonymous with physical addiction. Chein concluded that heroin has no universal addictive impact particularly if taken on less than a daily basis, and suggested that the emphasis of users on 'addiction' may be in part a defence-mechanism to rationalize their psychological involvement with the drug. Perhaps the fact that in New York City the heroin content of what is sold to the addict in the street is apparently so low as to be often almost negligible may have something to do with the ease with which some of Chein's subjects were able to move in and out of usage, although some experts have pointed out that where the heroin content is low, a greater number of injections may be taken to achieve the desired effect. What this finding does suggest is that opiates provide satisfactions which are sufficiently attractive to some people, with or without the iron grip of addiction, to maintain a cycle of personal involvement. And this may also explain why some people who have been accidentally addicted to morphine through medical use have been able to extricate themselves without further relapse, while many illicit users quickly become addicted with what seems to be deliberate intent. The *basis* of addiction may be biological – as the animal experiments would seem to indicate – but the individual's psychology may be very important in *reinforcing* the basic physical dependence. Thus, the withdrawal symptoms experienced early in opiate use are more tolerable than those experienced later, but if, as some authorities suggest, the personality that finds opiate use rewarding tends to be of the type that avoids unpleasant problems – the very reason for opiate use in the first place – then even mild withdrawal symptoms will be avoided by taking another dose, and thus the cycle is reinforced. Similarly, some addicts, even after being 'cured', have experienced a spontaneous recurrence of withdrawal symptoms when faced with difficult psychological strains.[30]

This leads us to the important question of the psychological basis of opiate use. If opiates act to alter the interpretation of pain in normal individuals, then they also act to reduce the level of anxiety and to artificially relieve tensions in some individuals whose ability to adapt to difficult circumstances may be limited. One medical study in 1948 concluded that "patients who have made a marginal degree of emotional adjustment to life, and then have begun to use drugs, lose some of their normal adaptive patterns of adjustment. This regression in personality represents the greatest danger of drug addiction."[31] The results of another study in New York suggested that personality "malfunctions" among delinquent youths were strongly related to drug addiction, although the authors of the study were careful to point out that the converse is not necessarily true: youths with access to opiates who exhibit personality disorders similar to those of addicted youths do not always, or even very often, become addicts themselves.[32] This view has been summarized by one writer, who suggests that the addict is

responding to personality problems of great complexity. The drug addict is a person with certain personality characteristics who happens to have selected this way of coping with his problems for a variety of reasons, of which he is usually unaware. Not the least of these reasons is his access to a social group in which drug use was both practised and valued.

He takes one drug rather than another because it provides satisfaction for him. Other people with exactly the same kind of personality substratum never become addicts and select other means of expression for their basis conflicts.[33]

Chein and his associates in New York maintained that all of their young addict subjects suffered from major, and deep-rooted, personality disorders. They were unable to maintain stable relationships with others; the male addicts (who appear to vastly outnumber female addicts everywhere in North America) had experienced great difficulty in assuming the aggressive masculine role which society demands of young men. They felt themselves to be failures and were easily frustrated, but they also found any form of frustration unbearable. While there was no single type of maladjustment associated with addicts, overt and incipient schizophrenia, delinquency-dominated and generally inadequate personalities were the main diagnoses.[34] What heroin offers to such personalities is an easy means of conflict resolution. All their daily problems are replaced by the single problem of obtaining the next dose. And with each injection, the tensions and anxieties which have been channelled into the all-encompassing craving for drugs are instantly, almost magically, dispelled and a state of deep, but temporary, psychic peace prevails.

People seek to maintain themselves in some sort of equilibrium with their environment. When the demands of the environment become overwhelming and an individual cannot adapt sufficiently without losing his identity, or his inner stability, then some new means of restoring equilibrium may be sought. The individual may begin re-interpreting the world in terms of his own inner needs and will thus begin to appear 'crazy' or 'schizophrenic' to outsiders. He may become aggressive and try to impose his own ideas on the environment and thus become known as 'criminal' or 'psychopathic'. He may try the familiar strategy of 'drowning his sorrows'. He may, especially if he comes from a middle-class background, seek professional help, whether psychiatric or medical. But there are many people in our society, especially at the lower income levels, who do not have access to expensive medical services, and who are not brought up to recognize their personal problems as being subject to professional aid, and who are thus ill-prepared to seek therapy in the socially-approved fashion. The disturbed young man or woman in an urban slum area may seek some form of self-therapy to resolve the explosive problems building up inside, and one possibility to which they may have relatively easy access is the illicit narcotics market, which flourishes within the urban slum environment. Some may find that opiates do nothing for them, and they will not continue to use them. But for some, the artificial resolution of conflicts which opiates offer will seem the answer to all their problems, and they will thus enter the long tunnel of addiction, arrest, relapse, re-arrest, and perhaps a lifetime of petty criminality to procure the necessary funds to buy their drugs.

This is the most common portrait of the drug addict. But such a portrait is by no means proven to be complete. It may fairly be said that too many investigators have begun their work with the assumption that addicts must be psychologically disordered and have then proceeded to find such disorders. Behavioral scientists have in recent years become more aware of what are known as *experimenter effects*, that is, the degree to which the expectations of the investigator help to determine his results.[35] Too few studies have employed such devices as blind interviews, in which the subject is not identified as an addict. Another problem is that all the studies have been based on subjects who are already officially known as addicts, usually through previous arrests: are the apparent personality disorders a cause or a result of the subjects' social position as losers and outcasts? It would be very interesting to see the results of tests done on addicts who are successful enough that they have not been arrested or otherwise identified. Perhaps an altogether different picture might emerge: after all, psychological testing of non-addicted criminal delinquents also shows a high rate of personality disorder, but it does not follow from this that *all* non-addicts are similarly unbalanced. Unfortunately, such tests would be extremely difficult to perform; the laws being what they are, no addict successful enough to evade the police is likely to volunteer to expose himself to identification through a long series of tests, regardless of the safeguards. The point here is that the law seriously interferes with the scope of scientific research into the true nature of a phenomenon which the law has already prejudged. But this prejudgment clearly was not based on a wide understanding of the phenomenon. Worse, attempts to gather sufficient information either to challenge or to affirm the wisdom of the law are themselves hampered by the same law.

The police maintain confidently that almost all the addicts are known, and it may well be that in the urban slum areas, the chances of evading arrest over an extended period of time may be very slim indeed. But even if we assume that the personality of the archetypal criminal addict of the slums has been adequately described, we have only dealt with one aspect of the addict personality, not with the phenomenon in its entirety. As we pointed out earlier, opiate addiction was relatively more common in the nineteenth century than today, and was not especially linked to slum areas, economically depressed groups, or to criminal elements. While it is clearly true that stiff anti-narcotics laws of the twentieth century have resulted in a tendency for addiction to be concentrated in urban slums, it is by no means clear that this is the only type of addiction now present in our society. In Canada, the Federal Government keeps statistics on three types of addicts: *criminal*, *medical* (those who have become accidentally addicted), and *professional* (mainly doctors with easy access to opiate supplies). These figures will be examined in detail in the next chapter, but the important point is that the possibility of official detection obviously varies from a high point with the criminal addicts, who are usually concentrated in areas where police surveillance is intense and who run a heavy risk of exposure through informers and undercover agents, to a lower point with 'respectable' and wealthier persons, with access either directly to drugs or to those persons, such as doctors, who do have such access. One study undertaken for the Presidential Commission on Law Enforcement in the United States included calculation of the number of individual doses of opiates which were medically administered in 1963 throughout the entire country. The somewhat startling result was that on an average, every man, woman and child had received five and one half legal doses in a single year.[36] Considering that many people never receive opiate medication, the number of legally prescribed doses per person receiving must be much higher. One may conclude either that fairly heavy medical opiate use need not always lead to addiction – which gives further evidence to the assumption that addiction is a much more complex process than has usually been assumed – or that there are many more opiate addicts than are officially known, which in turn indicates that many addicts may appear as relatively normal members of society.

It is the latter possibility which is especially interesting for it opens up one of the most important questions in the entire matter of drug addiction: to what extent are the alleged social and personal dangers of addiction the actual result of drug use itself and to what extent are they rather the result of the pre-existing social and psychological conditions of the addict? More importantly still, to what extent are they simply the result of the position into which a working-class slum-dwelling addict is forced by the laws against addiction? It is almost axiomatic in Parliament, in the courts, and in the media, that drug-addiction equals crime, prostitution, and human degradation. True, all these symptoms are associated with addiction, *where addiction is generally known by the police and studied by medical and social scientists.* But if more isolated, middle-class addicts have been able to escape detection, then it may be that many of these social evils are merely symptoms of the active legal repression of addicts rather than of addiction itself.

Consider the following problem: as an addict, you have a powerful demand for a particular good, heroin. There is, however, no legal supply. Moreover, zealous law enforcement, backed by tremendous punitive powers, makes the sale of heroin a risky affair. To compensate for such risk, the price is high, often astronomical. You are poor, and work opportunities are limited and low-paying. If you have been arrested before, your chances of getting any kind of steady job are almost non-existent. But if you cannot procure the necessary supply, you will become deathly ill. Where do you find the money? If you are a man, petty crime may be the means; if you are a woman, prostitution. In either case, peddling heroin to other addicts may be another answer. Deprived of a steady job and an acceptable social role, your life soon begins to centre around the one meaningful activity – buying and taking heroin. Forced to neglect your other needs to pay for your daily supply, you will probably become thin and unhealthy, and the dirty needle of your illegal hypodermic may give you infection. You will almost certainly be arrested a number of times, and your life will begin to seem sordid and futile – but the worse these feelings become, the more necessary heroin becomes to relieve such tensions. There is nowhere to go, and you no longer give a damn about your health or your appearance.

The middle-class opiate addict is in a very different position. If he has the financial means to keep his supply, which may come from a doctor within the context of medical therapy, there will be no need for him to become enmeshed in the dreary cycle of crime and arrest which is the lot of his working-class counterpart. Unfortunately, we do not know very much about such middle-class addicts here in North America – their numbers, their social and psychological characteristics, or their means of supply. What can be said is that they do not form an addict subculture, as is the case with slum addicts. One study was made of forty-seven physician addicts at the Fort Worth, Texas, Federal hospital, which concluded that the physician addict differs from the typical addict on a wide array of characteristics.[37] This is suggestive, but even here the subjects were already patients in a government institution. In Britain, until recently, addicts who obtained their minimum dose through private medical prescriptions seemed to have been quite different in character from the typical North American addict, and were often relatively unaware of other addicts. Many seemed to function more or less normally as productive citizens, despite their addiction.[38] The evidence cited earlier concerning the nature of opiate addiction in the nineteenth century confirms this observation, since many addicts seem to have been useful and creative members of society.

The unpleasant truth which must be faced is that we do not know a great deal about the essential nature of opiate addiction, or about its actual personal and social consequences – and one of the reasons we know so little is the legal status of narcotics. There is a crucial principle in contemporary physics, called Heisenberg's Uncertainty Principle, which states, very roughly, that at the level of subatomic particles, the attempt of the scientific observer to measure such particles will itself alter the state of the objects being measured; in other words, there is a point beyond which the human observer alters phenomena by the very action of observing them. There seems to be a somewhat similar mechanism at work in the problem of opiate addiction. The existence of strong laws against addiction has tended to change the phenomenon of addiction itself, and it becomes difficult to separate the properties of addiction from the consequences of legal repression.

This is not to say, of course, that the laws should necessarily be repealed, simply for the satisfaction of professors who want to investigate the problem in the most effective possible manner. But it is clear, on the one level, that a half century of anti-narcotics legislation has tended to transfer the problem from one of general social-economic distribution toward a much heavier concentration in crime-infested urban slums. On another level, it has led to a confusion of the endemic social and psychological diseases of slum-dwellers with the consequences of opiate addiction – a confusion which in many ways appears to be very misleading and always serves to add fuel to attempts to make legislation and penalties ever more severe.

But even if the most knowledgeable authorities cannot precisely describe the exact personal and social characteristics of opiate addiction, it is possible to separate the obviously false myths from reasonable observations. The unsettling truth on this point is that however little medical and social science may know, what *is* known constitutes sufficient ammunition to shoot down almost all the popular stereotypes of the drug addict, and with them much of the rationale of our anti-narcotics legislation. Let us examine some of these myths.

1. *The 'dope peddlar' myth.* Whenever the question of drug addiction arises in Parliament or comes to the considered attention of editorial writers, the evil 'dope peddlar' is sure to take a verbal beating. Innocent children are pictured as being ensnared by free samples which hook them forever, leaving them the continual victims of the peddlar's greed. This picture is hopelessly distorted on almost all counts. First of all, as we pointed out earlier, it is a fallacy that opiates are inherently attractive to the average person; in fact they are normally upsetting and unpleasant. Second, addiction is not something which immediately sets in with one injection – continuous daily use is necessary for a period, which would imply that novice users must be highly motivated. Third, the 'free sample' concept would be suicidal for the supplier; experienced addicts could seek out new suppliers and pretend to be interested non-addicts. Fourth, the hard reality of the addict subculture is that almost all peddlars are themselves addicts, who sell to feed their own habits. One can surmise that those at the top of the narcotics pyramid are smart enough not to be addicts themselves, but the 'big boys' are rarely caught because they probably never allow the goods to pass through their own hands. The weakest link in the chain of distribution is the addict in the street, and invariably it is he who is arrested. By striking at the 'peddlar', the law often does little but add to the already heavy legal burden on the addict himself.

The 'dope peddlar' myth is misleading, because it directs attention from the real problem. Like the Communist conspiracy myth, it creates a convenient bogey-man upon whom all our fears can be projected. "We are all happy here, it's only those outside agitators who are stirring up trouble: get rid of those Reds and you will get rid of all unrest." "Jail all those dope peddlars and the drug problem will disappear." As attractive as this may sound, it will not work. The fault, after all, is not in the stars but in ourselves. Jail all the peddlars and more will take their place, *because the demand for opiates will remain.*

The Presidential Crime Commission in the United States stated flatly that "there is no evidence from any study of initiation as a consequence of aggressive peddling to innocents who are 'hooked' against their will and knowledge . . . . The popular image of the fiendish peddlar seducing the innocent child is wholly false."[39] An official of the Ontario Department of Reform Institutions has also suggested that "there is no evidence which indicates that innocent, unwilling people are in any way dragged or forced into drug addiction."[40]

2. *Drug addicts are all criminals.* On one level this myth is true, for there are few addicts in Canada who are not breaking the law by buying illicit narcotics. But this, of course, begs the question. The real question is: to what extent are addicts criminals with regard to matters not directly related to their drug habits?

The most intensive study undertaken in Canada of opiate addiction, found that the typical Vancouver addict was an unskilled and unemployed worker who had been imprisoned for petty criminality, came in contact with addicts in prison, and left prison deeply caught up in the web of criminal associations and drug use.[41] It has been suggested that of drug addicts in Canada with criminal records, seventy-five per cent become addicts *after* the pattern of criminal behavior has already begun.[42] It has also been argued many times that the ordinary addict is forced into a life of crime to support his habit. These two perspectives are not necessarily contradictory, for *access* to narcotics is undoubtedly highest among the criminal elements of slum areas, but once addiction has set in, any escape from a life of petty crime becomes very much more difficult. It remains a matter of speculation as to whether the crime rate would be lowered significantly were addiction to disappear. It may well be that urban criminality is a structural problem of poverty in our society, of which drug addiction is merely a symptom.

What *can* be measured is the effect of addiction on the type of crime committed. The popular stereotype is the dope-crazed fiend, hopped-up to inhuman heights of violence and recklessness. Cocaine, which gives rise to short, euphoric bursts of energy, was once used

by criminals as a stimulant and it is possible that a confusion between it and heroin, also a white powder, led to heroin's present
reputation as an inducement to dangerous behavior.[43] The facts are
all the other way. Pharmacologically, the idea of anyone being
'hopped-up' on opiates, which are depressants, is nonsense. One
authority on addiction, has stated vividly that "both heroin and
morphine in large doses change drunken, fighting psychopaths into
sober, cowardly, non-aggressive idlers.[44] Another observer put it
this way.

> When they are
> in the street
> they pass it
> along to each
> other but when
> they see the
> police they would
> run some would
> just stand still
> and be beat
> so pity ful
> that they want
> to cry

This poem was written by Mary, age eleven, a resident of Harlem.[45]
The fact is that the crimes committed by junkies are likely to be
crimes against property rather than against persons, for the junkie is
primarily interested in money to feed his habit. Data compiled by the
Chicago police show that the number of arrests of addicts for violent
crimes against persons, such as rape and assault, was only a fraction
of the proportion of such arrests in the population at large.[46]

Nor is it any more sensible to argue that criminality is a symptom
of drug addiction, as such. Physician addicts and medical addicts are
usually associated with law-breaking only in regard to narcotics
laws. British addicts who obtain legal minimum doses at cost have
not been closely associated with crime. O'Donnell studied a sample
of 266 Kentucky addicts after release from prison. Of those who
received their drugs from a single doctor, there were almost no post-
release crimes. Among those who used several doctors, twenty-three
per cent had re-arrests. Those who combined medical and illicit
street sources showed a re-arrest rate of sixty-two per cent, and
among those whose supply was entirely from street peddlars,

seventy-two per cent returned to prison. O'Donnell suggests that drug use *per se* does not cause crimes, but that criminality is related to the source of drugs.[47]

3. *Addicts are sex maniacs.* Of all the myths surrounding opiate addiction this is certainly the most preposterous. In fact, it is the universal testimony of addicts that opiates depress and often eliminate sexual desire. Indeed the overall effects of opiates upon those who are addicted to them is to act as a *replacement* for the sexual drive. The only possible explanation for the myth of the dope-crazed sex fiend is that our society is so obsessed with sex that it must project its own suppressed fantasies onto scapegoats, for which role addicts are leading candidates.

4. *Drug addiction destroys morality.* It is obvious that the craving of an addict for his drug may be so total that all other considerations will be subordinated to the drive to obtain his supply, and in this sense it may be true that addiction tends to distort the moral judgments which an individual might normally make. But again, we face a confusion between addiction *per se*, and addiction within a repressive legal framework. The addict in the grip of a compulsion to obtain more drugs can be a dangerous individual, but only because his needs are being thwarted. Given a maintenance dose at cost, such compulsion may largely disappear, and the moral judgments of a normally-functioning individual are again possible. After all, people who are starving to death are apt to do things that they would never consider were they well-fed.

Since most known addicts come from a lower-class environment, and those who deal with them as agents of the state (police, social workers) tend to be more middle-class in background, there may be a certain degree of class bias in some of the judgments made. As one writer has stated

Little evidence has been adduced to show that the morality of the addict undergoes a significant modification as a result of his drug use.
It would appear, rather, that the addict, in arousing middle-class emotion by his drug use, brings the mores of his subculture into question. Rather than deal with the question of the morality of lower class patterns, the middle-class arbiters of the moral ethic label them a result of degenerate narcotics use.[48]

5. *Drug addiction causes physical degeneration.* Perhaps the most commonly held belief about addiction is that it is physically

self-destructive. There is no question that the addict experiencing withdrawal symptoms is a very sick individual, but such symptoms are caused by the absence of opiates, not by their presence. But what are the long-term effects of opiate *use*? Such a question is obviously crucial in any judgments concerning the dangers of drug addiction, and once again, the answer is incompatible with the accepted myth.

There seems to be little or no evidence that the continued use of opiates "causes permanent changes in the brain or central nervous system, or that it causes any changes except the body's greater tolerance of the drug."[49] Moreover, it appears that with addicts, behavior under the influence of opiates tends to be *more* 'normal' than behavior without opiates.[50] Addicts themselves agree that whatever euphoria opiates may have afforded in the early stages of their use, they later serve only to maintain normality and to avoid withdrawal sickness. This raises the important question of whether an opiate addict can function in a job. The U.S. Presidential Crime Commission found that there was no evidence of any correlation between addiction and industrial accidents, and also stated that there was clinical agreement that if addicts were given maintenance doses, no reduction of physical or mental task performance need occur.[51] Even more interesting was the testimony given by Dr. Lawrence Kolb to a U.S. Senate Committee a number of years ago. Dr. Kolb described some persons, including physicians, he had examined who were capable of useful work when addicted, but became hopelessly inadequate when 'cured'. Others were incompetent alcoholics until they switched their dependency from alcohol to morphine. They then achieved good industrial records.[52] The point is obviously not that opiates are good for you, but that for a particular type of person who lacks the ability to adjust to the demands of his environment, to whom anxieties are normally overwhelming, continuous use of some tension-reducing drug may be a means of adjustment. It may not be a very intelligent means, and it may not be in the addict's long-term interests, but his addiction must be understood within this context.

Everyone who has ever worked in a large organization will be familiar with the problem of the chronic alcoholic holding a job that he is no longer capable of fulfilling. Sometimes pathetic, sometimes obnoxious, the alcoholic is invariably useless because the means he employs to resolve his problems incapacitate him for the tasks he is supposed to perform. The case of the opiate addict is somewhat different, and in a sense, less socially wasteful, since his addiction may allow him to remain productive, *so long as his supply is assured.* One New York addict has recounted how he worked in an office where people discussed drug addicts and how he took part in the discussions, without anyone suspecting that he had any personal knowledge of drugs, even though he was in fact high on heroin. Drugs, he suggests, allow addicts to "get back into the routine, the cycle of things."

Give them the dope, they'll work eight hours a day, and you will never know the difference. Of course, after a while the effect of the heroin gives them a normal look. At first when you take dope, you're able to get high, you start getting sleepy; but after acquiring a habit you're just sick, and you need it just to become a normal human person. You can work and nobody knows the difference. I even used to work overtime.[53]

This is not to suggest that an addict will necessarily be able to work effectively if supplied with a maintenance dose. The personal inadequacies and disorders which led to drug use in the first place may preclude the individual from ever functioning normally. But from the point of view of social policy toward opiates, it should be understood that, in the words of one writer, "it appears far more likely that the addict responds to his weakness and ineffectiveness by using drugs rather than the reverse."[54]

It may thus be seen that the common myths about drug addicts do not stand up to close scrutiny. There seems to be little reason to fear the junkie as a menace comparable to the black plague; and there seems to be every reason to try to help addicts in the same way as help is offered to other sick persons. And yet the shocking truth is that instead of help, the addict has been offered rejection and persecution. Society has a supreme capacity to shape the individuals who belong to it, and a supreme indifference to the results of its policy. In medieval Europe, the Church declared that interest rates on loans were immoral. Christians thus sought out Jews as money-lenders – and then cursed them as Shylocks. Blacks in North American society were maintained forcibly in the role of menial labourers – and then characterized as obviously unfit for anything other than shoe-shining. Women are brought up from earliest childhood to be mothers and housewives – and then dismissed as being inferior to men in the work world. Drug addiction is declared to be a criminal activity, addicts are hunted down like criminals – and then in justification of these procedures it is explained that, after all, they act like criminals.

Sir John A. Macdonald cut right to the root of this form of social hypocrisy when, in regard to the French-speaking minority in Canada, he wrote, "treat them as a nation and they will act as a free people generally do – generously. Call them a faction and they become factious."[55] What is particularly disheartening about the treatment of drug addicts is that the mythology has so dehumanized the image of the addict that for many people compassion becomes very difficult. And yet what is it that makes those silent rituals behind locked doors, those personal, private acts with spoons, needles, eye-droppers and knotted towels, such a threat to our civilization and our social stability? What is it about someone injecting diluted heroin into a vein that should call forth such fulminations as that of the Democratic candidate for the United States Presidency in 1968: ". . . rioting, burning, sniping, mugging, traffic in narcotics, and disregard for the law are the advance guard of anarchy, and they must and they will be stopped." It is one thing to recognize opiate addiction as a *problem*, which it certainly is, but it is quite another to so encumber the problem with ill-founded moralism that the only solution which can eventually be contemplated is one of quasi-military annihilation.

It is difficult, if not impossible, to rationally explain the development of the dope-fiend myth and of its persistence in the face of almost all medical and scientific knowledge. But the fact remains that to the ordinary person, confronting drug addiction has about the same shock value as confronting public masturbation. The junkie having a fix is apparently playing out something too unsettling for the average person to contemplate with indifference. Perhaps a close look at the terrible poverty of the average junkie's life and the nightmare world of his anxieties and disorders is altogether too close to the average person's own fears and miseries. The myth is easier, and more comforting. By busting the junkie, we prove our own normality, just as children will inevitably gang up on any child who is weak or different, in a cruel and desperate attempt to demonstrate their own 'togetherness'. It is an old and sad story of human conduct – only the participants have changed.

It must be clear to anyone with an open mind that drug addiction is essentially a *medical* problem. Specialization may have its disadvantages but nobody has yet demonstrated that policemen, judges, and prison wardens are better qualified to solve medical problems than medical doctors. It is strange that North American society, which has elevated doctors to a very high level of prestige and of material award, should have decided that while they are competent to transplant hearts, they are not, generally, competent to deal with the problem of drug addiction; and that the legislatures and the courts must necessarily prescribe what is good and what is bad medical practice with regard to addiction. No one knows enough about addiction to state with confidence what cure is best, or indeed if there is any cure, but we do know enough to state with confidence that if one makes of a medical problem a criminal problem, one then ends up with two problems instead of one.

Footnotes

[1]Colin MacInnis, "Leaves of Grass," *Encounter*, vol. XXVIII, no. 4 (April, 1967), p. 67.

[2]Edith Hamilton, *Mythology* (New York, Mentor, 1953), p. 107.

[3]Robert Graves, *The Greek Myths* (Harmondsworth, Middlesex, Penguin Books, 1957) vol. I, pp. 89-96.

[4]DeRopp, *Drugs and the Mind, op. cit.*, p. 136.

[5]*Collected Writings of Thomas de Quincey*, David Masson, ed. (London, A. and C. Black, 1897), vol. III, p. 381.

[6]*Ibid.*, p. 400.

[7]Horace Ainsworth Eaton, *Thomas de Quincey: a Biography* (New York, Oxford University Press, 1936).

[8]Coleridge, "Kubla Khan".

[9]Quoted in Elisabeth Schneider, *Coleridge, Opium and Kubla Khan* (Chicago, University of Chicago Press, 1953), p. 318.

[10]*Ibid.*, p. 336.

[11]Alethea Hayter, *Opium and the Romantic Imagination* (London, Faber, 1968).

[12]Jean Cocteau, *Opium: The Diary of a Cure* (New York, Grove Press, 1957).

[13]Marie Nyswander, *The Drug Addict as a Patient* (New York, Grune and Stratton, 1956).

[14]*President's Commission on Law Enforcement, op. cit.*, p. 42; DeRopp, *op. cit.*, pp. 145-46.

[15]Isidor Chein *et al.*, *The Road to H: Narcotics, Delinquency, and Social Policy* (New York, Basic Books, 1964), p. 348.

[16]J. J. Lewis, *An Introduction to Pharmacology*, 3rd ed. (Baltimore, Williams and Wilkins, 1964), pp. 392-418.

[17]H. Isbell and W. White, "Clinical characteristics of addictions," *American Journal of Medicine*, vol. 14, no. 5 (May, 1953), p. 558.

[18]W. M. Davis and J. R. Nichols, "Physical dependence and sustained opiate-directed behavior in the rat," *Pharmacologia*, vol. III (1962), pp. 139-45.

[19]James R. Weeks, "Experimental Narcotic Addiction," *Scientific American* (March, 1964). Reprinted in Scientific American, *Psychobiology: The Biologi-*

cal Bases of Behavior (San Francisco, W. H. Freeman and Co., 1967), pp. 351-57.

[20]Quoted in Alfred Lindesmith, *The Addict and the Law* (Bloomington, Indiana, Indiana University Press, 1965), p. 23.

[21]DeRopp, *op. cit.*, pp. 150-54.

[22]David Ebin, ed., *The Drug Experience* (New York, Orion Press, 1961), p. 178.

[23]Isbell, *op. cit.*, pp. 72 and 74.

[24]David P. Ausubel, *Drug Addiction: Physiological, Psychological, and Sociological Aspects* (New York, Random House, 1958), p. 23.

[25]*Ibid.*, pp. 18-30.

[26]Chein, *op. cit.*, pp. 231-32.

[27]Helen M. Hughes, *The Fantastic Lodge: The Autobiography of a Girl Drug Addict* (Boston, Houghton Mifflin, 1961), p. 128.

[28]Alfred Lindesmith, *Opiate Addiction* (Evanston, Illinois, Principia Press, 1947). See also the same author's "Basic problems in the social psychology of addiction and a theory," in John O'Donnell and John C. Ball, eds., *Narcotic Addiction* (New York, Harper and Row, 1966), pp. 91-109.

[29]Chein, *op. cit.*, pp. 57-62.

[30]*Ibid.*, pp. 227-50.

[31]V. Vogel, H. Isbell, and K. Chapman, "Present status of narcotic addiction," *Journal of the American Medical Association*, vol. 138 (Dec. 4, 1948), p. 1999.

[32]D. Gerard and C. Kornetsky, *Adolescent Opiate Addiction: a Study of Control and Addict Subjects* (New York University, Research Center for Human Relations, 1955).

[33]Charles Winick, "Narcotics Addiction and its treatment," *Law and Contemporary Problems*, vol. 22, no. 1 (Winter, 1957).

[34]Chein, *op. cit.*, pp. 192-226.

[35]R. Rosenthal, *Experimenter Effects in Behavioral Research* (New York, Appleton-Century-Crofts, 1966).

[36]*President's Commission on Law Enforcement, op. cit.*, pp. 46-47.

[37]Michael J. Pescor, "Physician Drug Addicts," in J. A. O'Donnell and J. C. Ball, eds., *Narcotic Addiction* (New York, Harper and Row, 1966), pp. 164-67.

[38]Edwin M. Schur, *Narcotic Addiction in Britain and America: The Impact of Public Policy* (Bloomington, Indiana, Indiana University Press, 1962).

[39]*President's Commission on Law Enforcement, op. cit.*, p. 51.

[40]Frank Potts in *Canadian Journal of Corrections*, vol. I, no. 2, p. 41.

[41]George H. Stevenson, *Drug Addiction in British Columbia* (Vancouver, University of British Columbia, 1956).

[42]Potts, *loc. cit.*

[43]H. Isbell, "Historical development of attitudes toward opiate addiction in the United States," in S. M. Farber and H. L. Wilson eds., *Conflict and Creativity* (New York, McGraw-Hill, 1963), pp. 154-70.

[44]L. Kolb, quoted in D. M. Maurer and V. H. Vogel, *Narcotics and Narcotics Addiction*, 3rd ed. (Springfield, Illinois, Charles C. Thomas, 1967), p. 274.

[45]Quoted in Herbert Kohl, "Children writing: the story of an experiment," *New York Review of Books*, vol. VII, no. 8 (Nov. 17, 1966), p. 26.

[46]H. Finestone, "Narcotics and criminality," *Law and Contemporary Problems,* vol. XXII, no. 1 (Winter, 1957), p. 71.

[47]John O'Donnell, "Narcotic addiction and crime," *Social Problems,* vol. XIII (1966), pp. 374-84.

[48]William Butler Eldridge, *Narcotics and the Law: a Critique of the American Experiment in Narcotic Drug Control,* An American Bar Foundation Study, 2nd ed., rev. (Chicago, University of Chicago Press, 1967), pp. 19-20.

[49]Winick, *op. cit.,* p. 13.

[50]Nyswander, *op. cit.,* p. 61.

[51]*President's Commission on Law Enforcement, op. cit.,* pp. 54-55.

[52]DeRopp, *op. cit.,* pp. 148-49.

[53]Jeremy Larner and Ralph Tefferteller, eds., *The Addict in the Street* (Harmondsworth, Middlesex, Penguin Books, 1966), pp. 51 and 53.

[54]Eldridge, *op. cit.,* p. 22.

[55]Donald Creighton, *John A. Macdonald: the Young Politician* (Toronto, Macmillan, 1956), p. 227.

Opiates: Treating the Addict

Drug addiction is not, by any stretch of the imagination, a major health problem in Canada, on the scale of, say, alcoholism. In terms of statistical incidence, addiction would seem to be limited to about 0.02 per cent of the population. Moreover, the number of persons addicted to opiates appears to have been more or less stable over the past few years, with a slight upward trend in keeping with the general population increase. In 1962, for instance – the first full year under the Narcotic Control Act of 1961 – the Department of National Health and Welfare in Ottawa estimated that the total number of addicts in Canada was 3,576. In 1967 the estimate was 3,715.[1]

By contrast, it has been estimated that there were in 1924 some 9,000 addicts out of a total population of 9,200,000.[2] In other words, addiction has declined in both relative and absolute terms in the past forty or so years. Moreover, the geographical pattern of addiction indicates a shift in a steady westward direction. In the early 1930s Montreal was a focal point of addiction, with Toronto becoming the leader in the late 1930s. It was only after World War II that Vancouver became a centre of drug addiction. Today, addiction in Canada has become specifically a Vancouver problem, as may be seen in Table I.

This concentration becomes even more significant when it is considered that the government divides the addict population into three categories:

street or criminal addicts, including some addicts who have no criminal record but who are judged to have a "criminal background or criminal associations"

medical addicts, those who have become addicted through medical administration of opiates

	1962		1963		1964	
	No.	%	No.	%	No.	%
British Columbia	1,928(	53.9)	1,729(	51.5)	1,709(	51.0)
Ontario	995(	27.8)	971(	29.0)	1,009(	30.1)
Quebec	331(	9.3)	337(	10.0)	337(	9.6)
Prairies	266(	7.4)	267(	8.0)	267(	7.8)
Maritimes	56(	1.6)	51(	1.5)	51(	1.5)
Canada	3,576(	100.0)	3,355(	100.0)	3,352(	100.0)

	1965		1966		1967	
	No.	%	No.	%	No.	%
British Columbia	1,906(	53.3)	2,068(	57.6)	2,183(	58.8)
Ontario	1,033(	28.9)	953(	26.5)	958(	25.8)
Quebec	330(	9.2)	280(	7.8)	258(	6.9)
Prairies	259(	7.2)	251(	7.0)	275(	7.1)
Maritimes	45(	1.3)	40(	1.1)	41(	1.1)
Canada	3,573(	100.0)	3,592(	100.0)	3,715(	100.0)

Table I.   Estimated total number of addicts in Canada, 1962-67.

Source: Dept. of National Health and Welfare.

professional addicts, those who have daily access to opiates, such as doctors and nurses.

Names of known addicts are deleted from the latter two categories after five years without record of further drug involvement, and from the first category after ten years. In 1967 there were 231 recorded medical addicts, 149 professional addicts, and 3,335 criminal addicts. Medical and professional addicts are not concentrated in British Columbia, but are instead distributed fairly evenly throughout the country. In the criminal addict category, however, British Columbia's concentration is remarkable. Although only one out of every ten Canadians lives in B.C., two out of three criminal addicts are residents of that province, most of them apparently living in the Vancouver metropolitan region. Among males in the age group twenty-five to thirty-four, there are 424 criminal addicts per 100,000 population in British Columbia, as compared to only 18 per 100,000 population in all other provinces.[3] In 1961 the Federal

Minister of Justice, Mr. Davie Fulton, startled his fellow members of Parliament by pointing out that there was one criminal addict for every 390 residents of Vancouver as compared to one for every 5,700 in Canada as a whole.[4]

It is not clear why such a heavy concentration has taken place. There is no comparable west coast concentration in the United States, where New York and Chicago are major centres of addiction. Although the Canadian government first became aware of addiction problems with regard to the Chinese opium-smokers in British Columbia earlier in the century, the present addict population is almost exclusively non-Asian in ethnic origin.[5] Moreover there appears to be evidence that the narcotics traffic in Canada moves from the east to the west coast, so that even the geographical proximity of British Columbia to Asian sources of supply cannot be used as an explanation. We are left with the somewhat inadequate suggestion that the mild climate of the west coast may have attracted slum addicts, whose marginal economic status makes their lives in Toronto or Montreal too harsh. In any event, the Vancouver concentration is an essential demographic fact about drug addiction in Canada; any governmental attempts to deal with the problem thus have to be undertaken jointly by the Federal government and the British Columbia provincial government.

Of the known criminal addict population in 1967, 68 per cent were male and only 32 per cent female. Less than 1 per cent were under twenty years of age; 29 per cent were between twenty and twenty-nine; 31 per cent were between thirty and thirty-nine; 18 per cent between forty and forty-nine; after age fifty the figures drop considerably. 22 per cent of the addicts were listed as unskilled laborers, 12 per cent as being in service occupations, 8 per cent skilled labor, 6 per cent in national resources work, and 5 per cent were prostitutes; the largest percentage for occupation (30 per cent) was in the category of "unknown". Where the drug of addiction could be identified, heroin was the over-whelming favorite (71 per cent).[6]

The statistics given up to now have been based mainly on information gathered by the Department of National Health and Welfare. These statistics are the best available, but one must nevertheless express certain misgivings. It would seem to be extremely doubtful that *all* addicts are known to the government, particularly in regard to professional and medical addicts and to those from middle-class backgrounds with financial means.[7] Second, the means whereby the statistics are gathered, largely through criminal records, may bias some of the findings. For example, the finding that in 1967 less than 1 per cent of the criminal addict population was under twenty years of age, would seem to indicate that Canadian addicts start later in life than American addicts. It is, however, possible that the teenage incidence may be higher than the figures indicate as the longer a person is addicted the more his chances of being arrested increase; thus an addict starting out in his late teens might not be identified until his twenties. Another problem is that of older addicts whose names are carried forward year to year but who might have quit drugs in the meantime. Moreover, a relapse to drug use may be only an isolated event within a longer period of abstinence;[8] however, any unfavorable report on an addict will lead to his name being kept for a further ten years on the official list. These rather speculative criticisms are made not to condemn the Department of Health and Welfare, which is undoubtedly doing the best possible job under the circumstances, but rather to point out the need for more first-hand investigations of the addict subculture in Canada. Dr. George Stevenson provided such a study in the mid-1950s, although it has never received the circulation that it deserves. Now, over a decade later, more such studies, employing the most rigorous methods of social science, are very much needed before one can speak with any real confidence about the phenomenon of drug addiction in Canada. As in so many other areas of study one must now rely largely on American models to understand Canadian problems.

Whatever large gaps exist in our present knowledge of addiction are small indeed when compared to the almost complete ignorance that reigned when the decision was first made to set out on the road to a legislative, rather than a medical, solution to addiction. It is a curious accident of history that the original architect of our narcotics laws was that quintessential Canadian, Mackenzie King. In 1907, King, then a young Deputy Minister of Labour, was appointed a Royal Commissioner to investigate anti-Oriental riots in Vancouver, and was shocked to discover two claims for losses put forward by opium manufacturers. King then undertook a personal investigation, which included visits to opium dens and purchasing a package of opium across the counter of a store, and produced a report, "On the Need for Suppression of the Opium Traffic in Canada," which formed the basis for the *Opium and Drug Act of 1908*,[9] which prohibited all sales of opium. When the Minister responsible for the legislation tried to explain its provisions to the House of Commons, he was shouted down by the Opposition members, not out of partisanship, but because they preferred to pass the bill without having to bother examining its contents.[10] The following year King was sent to represent Canada at the International Opium Commission in Shanghai. He was sent because of his special knowledge, although, as one of his biographers significantly remarks, "even the most charitable could never have described King as an expert. The truth was that the Canadian service did not contain anyone qualified to challenge King's knowledge, such as it was, on the subject of opium . . . . In the country of the blind the one-eyed man was king."[11] The truth was also that at that time nobody anywhere knew very much about the mechanisms of addiction. Under such circumstances it was all too easy to assume that one could simply get rid of the problem by passing a law against it.

When it became apparent that the problem was not disappearing, the response was always to pass more legislation and to strengthen existing laws. There were other factors at work that also contributed to the reliance on punitive legislation. The decisions of successive International Opium Conventions, to which Canada was a party, was one such factor. Another was the extent to which Canada was perforce caught up in the internal dynamics of American attempts to deal with opiates. In 1914 the tough *Harrison Act* was passed in the United States, an Act that formed the basic legal structure for the ambitious American attempt to eradicate addiction by means of the criminal sanction, which has continued up to the present. The U.S. Narcotics Bureau, under Mr. Harry Anslinger (who recently retired) is a classic study of a bureaucratic agency that attempts to ensure its continued existence by the creation of a sympathetic environment within which to operate. This it has achieved by the distribution of information favorable to its policies, and, much more objectionably, by the active suppression or attempted discrediting of information unfavorable to its policies.[12] Strengthened by various court decisions and judical interpretations, the *Harrison Act* has proved to be a very successful instrument for the separation of the drug addict from the doctor who could most help him. As early as 1920, the influence of the American system could be felt in Canada when N. W. Rowell, the Minister responsible for the passage of a number of amendments to the *Opium and Drug Act* of 1908, put forward the *Harrison Act* as a major reason for stiffening Canadian laws.[13]

In the early 1920s a well-known Canadian began a personal crusade against the traffic in opiates. Judge Emily Murphy, an Edmonton magistrate and popular writer, had been deeply shaken by the number and desperation of the drug addicts whom she saw before her almost daily in court. A series of articles in *MacLean's Magazine* was followed in 1922 by the publication of *The Black Candle*,[14] a book that found a wide readership not only in Canada but in other countries as well, and that caused a good deal of public pressure to be put on both Federal and provincial governments to take stronger measures against illicit drug use. As a direct result of this book, "provincial Departments of Justice, in many instances, circularized the magistrates within their jurisdiction urging penalties that were more severe."[15] The tenor of Judge Murphy's views can be gained from her assertion that "unless the forces of civilization strangle the (drug) Rings – choke them to death, the Rings are going to choke civilization."[16] Although sympathetic to the plight of the white Anglo-Saxon addict, her concern was somewhat marred by an apparent belief that opiate addiction was a plot on the part of some Orientals and Negroes to destroy the ascendancy of the white race, and she used the issue of the opium traffic to suggest that Orientals be excluded from the country. "It is hardly credible that the average Chinese pedlar has any definite idea in his mind of bringing about the downfall of the white race, his swaying motive being probably that of greed, but in the hands of his superiors, he may become a powerful instrument to this very end."[17] There can be little doubt that Judge Murphy's writings did much to shape public opinion on the question of the proper policy toward drug addiction.

The first major change in the direction of Canadian law did not come until the passage of the *Narcotic Control Act* of 1961. Symbolically this Act was introduced jointly by the Minister of Justice and the Minister of Health and Welfare. The legislation similarly has two faces: on the one side, stern retribution, and on the other, medical help. For the first time, *addiction* itself has been recognized as a *medical* problem and provision for treatment written into the Act. But at the same time the 1961 legislation also includes many of the punitive features of the old law, although with more judicial discretion. One prominent critic of the American approach to addiction has contrasted the Canadian approach favorably to that of his own country, commenting that "Canada, which has long followed a system similar to that of the United States, appears to have found it unsatisfactory."[18]

The Act includes under the category of *narcotics* not only opium, morphine, heroin and other opiates, but also cocaine, marijuana, and a wide array of synthetic drugs. There are five separate offences involved in the Act – unauthorized possession of any narcotic, trafficking, possession for the purpose of trafficking, the unauthorized importing or exporting of any narcotic, and the unauthorized cultivation of the opium poppy or marijuana. Simple possession carries a maximum penalty of seven years imprisonment; trafficking or possession for trafficking carries a maximum of life imprisonment; importing and exporting carries a maximum of life and a mandatory minimum of seven years; unauthorized cultivation can bring a maximum of seven years imprisonment.[19] With the exception of the offence of importing and exporting, one important break with previous Canadian legislation, and with American practice, is the avoidance of mandatory minimum penalties. A Senate Committee that investigated the narcotics traffic in the 1950s had recommended that mandatory minimums be imposed on trafficking offences, but instead the Government opted for an increased maximum (life imprisonment) but with complete judicial flexibility in fixing sentences. American state legislatures have in recent years gone to extreme lengths in setting high minimum sentences without the possibility of parole; such an attempt to eliminate any judicial discretion is a counterpart to American attempts to eliminate any medical discretion on the part of doctors in the treatment of addicts. Happily, the Canadian government has seen fit to move in exactly the opposite direction. It is on this basis that young marijuana users have not been sent for long terms in the penitentiary without hope of parole as has occurred in some parts of the United States.

Greater flexibility in sentencing is one liberal aspect of the 1961 legislation; the other is in the provisions for medical treatment for addicts. The Act envisions two rigidly separated approaches to the addict and the non-addict narcotics offender. If a defendant is shown to be an addict he may be sentenced to "custody for treatment for an indeterminate period, in lieu of any other sentence that might be imposed for the offence of which he was convicted."[20] A person so sentenced has the right of appeal, as well as being eligible for parole. If released under parole, a first offender will be subject to supervision for ten years, and a second offender for an indefinite period.

Central to the implementation of this part of the Act is the creation of a pioneer treatment centre under provincial auspices at Matsqui, British Columbia. Similar centres are planned for Ontario and Quebec.

The recognition that the addict, as such, is a medical problem as much or more than he is a criminal problem is a very hopeful step. The fact that even an addict convicted of trafficking will be given treatment instead of prison is a valuable blow at the misleading myth of the dope-peddler. There are, however, other aspects of the 1961 Act that give cause for disquiet. One is the provision for preventive detention for non-addicted traffickers convicted of a second offence. The concept of preventive detention, at least for sexual offenders, is now coming under fire by the present government through the *Criminal Law Amendment Act* passed by the House on May 14th, 1969.

Another aspect that raises serious questions of individual liberty is contained in sections 7 and 8 of the 1961 Act. These sections require a defendant accused of possession of a narcotic to first prove to the Court that his possession was authorized under the Act. If he fails to prove this point the onus is once more put on him to prove that he was not in possession for the purpose of trafficking. In other words, the traditional principle of Anglo-Saxon jurisprudence, that a defendant is presumed innocent until proven guilty by the state, has been reversed. Under the *Narcotic Control Act* a defendant is in fact considered guilty until he himself proves to the state that his is *not* guilty. The burden of proof is shifted from the court to the defendant. Such an extraordinary procedure is presumably based on two premises: (1) narcotics represent such a endemic danger to society that extreme measures become necessary; (2) as there are normally no injured victims giving evidence against defendants in narcotics cases, the police task of preparing a case is so difficult that radically different procedures are required. The second premise is undoubtedly true, but it also manages to suggest that the offence in question may not be as grave as the first premise would indicate. Moreover, if the second part of the 1961 Act recognizes addiction as a medical problem, why the pressure to adopt procedures that are not allowed even in such grave criminal offences as murder? In fact it would appear that the courts have somewhat

modified the impact of the burden-of-proof provisions by interpreting them to mean that the onus is on the accused to adduce
evidence that will be sufficient to raise a reasonable doubt in the
mind of the judge.[21] Nevertheless the argument raised by Mr. Paul
Martin during debate on the Act, that the burden-of-proof provision
is contrary to the Bill of Rights, would seem to be justified.[22]

Similar objections can be raised to section 10, which provides for
special Writs of Assistance to be issued to named persons allowing
them "at any time, to enter any dwelling house and search for
narcotics."[23] Officers are further empowered to seize any object
that they feel may constitute evidence,[24] and to "break open any
door, window, lock, fastener, floor, wall, ceiling, compartment,
plumbing fixture, box, container or any other thing."[25] A vehicle
"that has been proved to have been used in any manner in connection with the offence" may be forfeited to the Crown.[26] Special
narcotics agents have thus been armed with warrants that allow
them to break into any house at any time and to wreak considerable
havoc in a search for narcotics. This power has taken on a somewhat
sinister aspect in regard to marijuana offences; this development will
be discussed in the next chapter. But the dangers of search and
seizure powers can be seen in the recent case of a Vancouver suspect
who died following an attempt by police to force him to disgorge
a quantity of narcotics he had swallowed. As one legal authority has
suggested, the problem of police brutality, "which so often accom-
panies search and seizure and the use of writs of assistance . . .
lowers the dignity of law enforcers and their own sense of that dignity. It may lead in time to a deadening insensitivity to the very
values which the policeman is dedicated to preserving."[27] The potential for harassment of individuals is also dangerous because the same
homes may be repeatedly entered and searched without recourse on
the part of the occupants. The revered tradition of one's home being
one's castle is thus turned into an empty joke by such legislation.
Canadians might do well to ask themselves if they really approve of
such extraordinary police powers. The point is not whether, or to
what extent, the police actually misuse these powers, but rather
that the statutory allowance for potential abuse ought to be very
carefully scrutinized. After all, it is human beings who make the
laws, enforce the laws, and break the laws. There is, to put it in the
most careful terms, no ironclad assurance that the worst aspects of
human nature will be found only in the latter category.

Putting aside these and similar misgivings about the punitive aspects of the *Narcotic Control Act*, we might now return to a consideration of some of the implications of its provisions for treatment. It cannot be overemphasized how important the treatment concept is, if only symbolically, as signifying an ideological break from the basic philosophy of a half-century of punitive narcotics laws. It is by no means obvious, however, that the 1961 approach promises, in terms of its specific content, any ultimate solution to the problem of drug addiction.

It is all too commonly believed that a 'cure' for addiction means simply that the addict quits using drugs. In the previous chapter we endeavored to demonstrate that a complex interaction of physiological, psychological, pharmacological, sociological, and criminological factors come together to make up the addiction syndrome, and, just as important, how many factors are not even identified or properly understood. Simple withdrawal from drugs may in fact remove a key element in a complicated personal equilibrium. Without dealing with the underlying causes of drug use, that is, without a careful attempt to make possible a personal equilibrium *without* the prop of drug use, a 'cure' may turn out to do more harm than good. As one commentator has suggested: "It is not enough to remove the patient from drug use if thereafter he suffers intensely from emotional disturbances, maladjustment, and disorientation from his social community. Substitution of one illness for another hardly seems to merit the term 'cure'."[28] Drugs have become the addict's means of adaptation. Unless other patterns of adaptation are successfully substituted, relapse to drug use will be inevitable.[29]

Canadian law points to an exclusively hospital-centred approach to the problem, based on legal compulsion. Unfortunately, experience with narcotics hospitals in the United States, at Lexington, Fort Worth, and Riverside Hospital in New York have not been encouraging, to say the least. In the past, patients at these centres have tended to be voluntary; despite this fact, the relapse rate of former patients is incredibly high, being variously estimated at between seventy-five and ninety-five per cent.[30] One author has suggested flatly that such statistics "tell the stark story of the basic failure of the hospital centered approach in dealing with the problems of drug addiction."[31] One problem encountered by such hospitals is that addicts use them as a stage in the development of their addiction. The tolerance mechanism means that the addict must procure more and more drugs to produce the same results. Eventually complete withdrawal may become necessary to get the habit back to manageable proportions. 'Cures', and relapses, may in this sense only be reinforcements to the general pattern of addiction.[32] Another factor working against the success of such hospitals is that the addict subculture is simply transferred into an institutional setting: drugs often dominate all talk, and thus continue to hold sway over the consciousness of the patients.[33] In the course of his stay, a patient may meet a number of connections that he can call upon later.

Despite the discouraging record of such hospitals, California, New York, and Massachusetts have adopted programs of compulsory civil commitment of addicts. These programs would seem to differ from the Canadian plan on at least two points. First, they do not replace conventional criminal sanctions, but instead seem directed toward taking off the streets addicts who have not already been so removed by criminal sentences. Second, the programs seem designed more to protect the public from the alleged dangers of addicts than to help the addicts themselves. The major criticism of civil commitment plans is that they represent an unreasonable deprivation of the individual's liberty without promising any solution to the problem.[34]

The Canadian approach is much more patient-oriented, and the persons involved in the Matsqui institution are obviously aware of the complex problems associated with addiction. The law itself foresees at least a ten-year supervision of a patient after he leaves the hospital. All is not well however. R. St.J. Macdonald of the University of Toronto Law Faculty has commented somewhat unfavorably on the potential of the British Columbia centre.

Matsqui . . . has all the earmarks of being another Lexington. It is too far away from the downtown metropolitan area and thus runs the risk of not being able to base an effective follow-up program. It may impress less than desirable attitudes upon its own treatment team, which is forced to live in a comparatively isolated community. It is too large, and its over-all orientation continues to be punitive rather than curial. The treatment context is just not right . . . . All in all, Matsqui may not be too successful. Lexington and Fort Worth have long demonstrated that, irrespective of length of commitment, the relapse rate is more than 75 per cent. Merely to get an addict off the street and into a Lexington type institution is not the answer. On the other hand, Matsqui is only a beginning, and one hopes that the experience gained from its operation will be taken into account when the government builds its projected units in Ontario and Quebec.[35]

One factor that cannot be overlooked, and that may limit the effectiveness of any such centre, is that the very deprivation of liberty and the compulsory immersion of a person within an all-encompassing institution may often make the patient feel as if he is merely an object and will thus effectively block the essential participation by the patient in his own development.[36] On the other hand, a drug addict is a person who is already enslaved to a drug, which has led some authorities to suggest that "only the most consistent type of coercion should be expected to work. By this, one does not imply that punishment, as such, is desirable, but that certain conditions of restriction of freedom may be required to assist in the establishment of motivation."[37] Obviously a very delicate and infinitely painstaking balance must be struck between these two poles.

One organization that has attempted to maintain this balance is Synanon, a group of self-contained communities of ex-addicts in the western United States, which are unofficial and unregulated but which appear to have achieved a far better record of cures than the government agencies. There is a Synanon-type halfway house now established in Vancouver with indirect government help through the services of the Company of Young Canadians. A good deal of coercion seems to be employed, but it is exercised through the dynamics of group interaction rather than through a rigid authority structure. At the centre of the Synanon approach is the group therapy session, where participants relentlessly probe each others' weaknesses.[38] Critics have, however, pointed out that few of the ex-addicts cured by Synanon ever return to the outside community; moreover, there is no encouragement given by Synanon to re-enter the everyday world.[39] "Synanon is the greatest addiction of all," say some of its members, and it clearly is possible that the protective little community has become an alternative dependency to dependency-prone personalities.

One group that split off from Synanon (most unamicably, on both sides) and does attempt to return members to the community outside is Daytop, in New York. Like Synanon, Daytop stresses the addict's responsibility for his own condition, and *stupidity* rather than illness as the cause of addiction.[40] Unfortunately, Daytop has recently been shaken by a vicious internal upheaval.[41] It seems that

Synanon-type organizations that stress group cohesion are peculiarly vulnerable to destructive internal struggles.

Both the strength and the weakness of Synanon and Daytop reflect one essential fact that must be taken into consideration when discussing 'cures'. Drug addiction in North America does not for the most part operate among isolated individuals, but within an addict subculture. Synanon and Daytop attempt to utilize this subculture as an instrument of change by setting up a life situation in which the internal dynamics of group interaction re-orient the goals of this subculture away from drugs toward a new direction. In a civilization like our own, which is characterized by conflicting values and widespread social alienation, it is possible that some of the appeal of drugs to particularly weak and vulnerable persons is the opportunity to join a subculture in which the essentially totalitarian need for drugs resolves all conflicts and doubts into a single, relentless all-encompassing community-wide activity and life-style. The addict thus finds himself a member of a community, of sorts, joined with others not unlike himself in a common goal: the acquisition of drugs. Synanon's use of this basic social unit is both clever and dangerous; thus its very failure to return members to the community at large is a sign of how successful its methods have been. Whether or not such methods suit the needs of the society outside is something else again.

The institutional method, such as that of Matsqui or Lexington, tends to incorporate some of the less desirable aspects of the addict subculture without using it beneficially in the way Synanon does. Addicts are concentrated together in an institution with the result that the old values are perpetuated, especially in view of the rigid 'we-they' dichotomy inevitable in an authoritarian environment.

It has been the universal finding of investigators that deviant subcultures tend to reinforce the deviant values of the individual member. Short of the adoption of a Synanon approach – which has its own dangers, as already pointed out, and which, moreover, must be a matter for private, grass-roots iniative among the addicts themselves – it seems fairly obvious that if the country is really serious about dealing with addiction, the place to begin is with the addict subculture. It does not seem unreasonable to suggest that a prime aim of legislation should be to remove as many addicts as possible from the subculture that sustains and reinforces their dependence on drugs. But the *Narcotic Control Act*, in both its punitive and its treatment aspects, tends to support the continued existence of the subculture. The addict in the street must turn to the subculture that organizes the distribution and sale of the drugs he needs, as no other source is normally available. But treatment within a compulsory setting does not necessarily alter the values of the group to which he belongs.

O'Donnell has described the evolution of drug addiction patterns in Kentucky in terms relevant to our argument. Before the passage of the *Harrison Act* in 1914, there was no addict subculture in Kentucky, as drugs could be purchased legally. Following 1914 a subculture arose to meet the need for drug distribution. After 1940 the subculture failed to provide a steady supply, and some addicts were able to establish a relationship with a physician who would provide them with a stable source. The subculture then withered away, and addiction seems to have generally diminished in the state. O'Connell comments that this pattern might

account for the fact that today narcotic addiction is almost entirely a metropolitan problem; relatively few addicts are known in smaller cities, towns and villages, where they used to be numerous. Similar considerations do not apply in metropolitan areas, where the illicit market has long been the major source of narcotics, and where the drug subculture still provides an effective solution to the problem of obtaining narcotics.[42]

Lady Frankau, a British doctor treating drug addicts, has described her experience in the treatment of some fifty Canadian addicts who fled punitive Canadian laws and sought help in Britain. Lady Frankau's methods involve first of all supplying the addict with a steady job and a maintenance dose so as to eliminate any contact between the addict and the local drug subculture. Initial psychotherapeutic treatment precedes any attempt at drug withdrawal. When the patient has established a good relationship with the doctor and a degree of stability and integration into normal community life, a process of gradual withdrawal is begun. The results appear to be far superior to the general treatment record of addicts in Canada.[43] What is important for our purposes here is that a key element in the Frankau program is the isolation of the individual addict from the addict subculture.

The British system of treating narcotics, that is, the administration of maintenance doses by physicians to individual patients was a clever attempt to eliminate the drug subculture. The theory was that if every existing addict could purchase his required dosage from a doctor, the black market would disappear and no new addicts would be created. Eventually addiction would simply fade away, as existing addicts either died or gave up drugs. Like most neat theories about human behavior, this has not in fact turned out to be very consistent with reality. Over-prescription led to a surplus that was then re-sold by addicts; under-prescription gave rise to a demand that the black market hastened to fill. And then in the past few years, an alarming rise in the number of addicts, particularly in the under-twenty age group, has completely changed the nature of the addiction problem in Britain. Now the British government is endeavoring to treat addicts at special centres, and the British public, which for years was relatively unconcerned with the tranquil drug scene, is as deeply alarmed about the 'dope menace' as the North American public.

The 'British system' has often been put forward as a panacea for the drug problem. As a panacea it has already proved to be a failure. But we need not deal always in absolutes. In fact so long as we search for final solutions we are bound to be frustrated. A cartoon I recall seeing in a magazine a number of years ago illustrates this point vividly. Two very perplexed businessmen were sitting in a car on a rough country road. An old farmer was leaning on a pitchfork saying, "You know, come to think of it, I don't think there's *any* way you can get to Chicago from here." The practical, optimistic, problem-solving North American mind rebels at this impertinence: there *must* be a road to wherever you want to go. But it may well be that the Final Solution to drug addiction is a mythical city, and to search for mythical cities may lead us far, far away not only from realistic policies but from ourselves, as human beings.

The North American attempt to outlaw opiate use by means of the criminal sanction rests on the essentially Utopian belief that the State can make man good, whether he wants to be good or not. If the British theory has not succeeded in eliminating addiction, neither has the American theory. It is, in fact, preposterous to believe that law enforcement, no matter how widespread and no matter how zealous, will ever be able to wholly stop supplies of heroin and morphine from entering the country and from being circulated within the country. As Eldridge has concisely put it:

Total elimination of access to drugs through suppression of smuggling, illicit traffic, and diversion from legitimate channels must be recognized as an unrealistic, impossible, and visionary goal. Therefore, to state the . . . proposition as if it were a complete answer does nothing but delude the public. Strict law enforcement can cut down severely on the amount of drugs coming into the country, but what will happen to the traffic which does get through?[44]

It is in this light that we must examine proposals for the administration of maintenance doses by licensed physicians. For, as the author of the New York Academy of Medicine's 1955 proposal for narcotics clinics to dispense drugs told a U.S. Senate Committee hearing, "We are simply advising a different method of distribution . . . every addict gets his drugs right now . . . why not let him have his minimum requirements under licensed medical supervision, rather than force him to get it by criminal activities, through criminal channels?"[45]

If we accept the idea that neither proscription nor prescription will eliminate drug addiction – and all the empirical evidence would seem to support this point – we can then recognize the existence of very deep-seated causes of addiction with which mere legislation is essentially powerless to deal. True, not all countries have opiate addicts, as such. There are, for example, only a tiny handful in France; it is, however, not without significance that France has the worst alcoholism problem of any country in the Western world. Where opiates have become part of the popular drug culture, opiate addiction is one symptom of underlying social malaise; where opiates are not well known, other addictions may serve the same function. The specific substances involved may not even be all that important, for medical studies of various addicts have time and again found evidence of considerable interchange of many drugs within the same personal pattern of addiction. What is important is the seared and twisted condition of life that drives people inward toward the endless, issueless short-circuiting of the human organism that any compulsive addiction must become. Reformers and liberals may rail against the continuous insult that addicts offer to visions of human perfection, but so long as addiction, in the sense of sticking needles into arms, is approached as a problem to be solved in complete isolation, then all attempts at reform solutions are almost certainly doomed. Of course, if poverty were eradicated and society restructured so that meaningful social action and participation were made possible for everyone, the compulsion toward addiction might wither[46] – but that is another story, and merely to state these preconditions is to demonstrate how far we are from achieving them.

It has been pointed out earlier that a fundamental reason for widespread opiate addiction in the nineteenth century was that medical science did not generally understand basic disease processes; physicians were only able to relieve symptoms – with remedies heavily laced with opiates – which often did little to cure the actual disease itself, but left the patients addicted to the drug that relieved their distressing symptoms. Today, of course, the aim of most medical treatment is to view unpleasant symptoms as warning signs and to proceed to treat the underlying disease or physiological process at work. It may be helpful to view the entire question of the social treatment of drug addiction as an analogy to the growth of medical science: addiction is not a *disease in itself*, but rather a *symptom* of much more complex underlying factors. Instead of taking this symptom as a helpful warning sign and then attempting to discover what factors are involved in the overall disease pattern, we have only tried to suppress the symptoms. When the symptoms fail to disappear, however, the answer is to take more doses of the original medicine, with the result that we have gradually become 'hooked' – on punitive law enforcement. Perhaps the 1961 *Narcotic Control Act*, with its provisions for medical treatment, may be the first tentative stages of a withdrawal process, hopefully without too many relapses along the way. But as with withdrawal from narcotics, this will only be an isolated step. Much more important is the coming to grips with the complex problems that underlie the existence of addictions in our society.

Nobody, to be sure, has the complete answer to the problem. But it cannot be overemphasized that it is not necessary to have an exact blueprint of an alternative plan in order to confront the existing system. I would be most suspicious of anyone claiming to possess such a blueprint as probably being just as dangerous as those who maintain that the existing system is a complete answer. The problem is not to construct an abstract solution to a set of concrete problems, but to construct a concrete situation within which concrete answers are most likely to emerge. By this I mean that every effort should be made to ensure that all possible avenues be left open to exploration. It is the essence of science that the *content* of future discoveries cannot be predicted; adherence to the scientific *method* of free inquiry, however, may be thought to ensure an ever-deepening knowledge of natural phenomena. Things are not, of course, all that clear cut with regard to human phenomena, but the principle remains a good one. What is essential is that the way be opened to experimentation and innovation in the investigation of drug problems.

At the very centre of any such innovative approach must lie the elimination of all the legal barriers that separate the drug addict from the medical doctor.

Exactly what constitutes good medical practice with regard to addiction should not be defined by legislative bodies, nor by the police. Alcoholics and sexual deviates offend against the common morality of society; yet doctors are free to treat such people as they see fit – why then must the State intervene so drastically between the addict and his doctor?

Already some results are coming in from the interaction of doctor and patient. We have already noted the success of Lady Frankau in Britain. Dr. Marie Nyswander and Dr. Vincent Dole, both of New York, have been achieving a good record of cures employing what is known as *methadone maintenance therapy*. This involves the daily administration of methadone, which eliminates the craving for opiates. An independent evaluation of their program[47] has indicated that after two years eighty-five per cent of the patients are employed or in school, as opposed to only twenty-eight per cent at the time they began treatment. Methadone treatment is now being used by the Narcotic Addiction Foundation of British Columbia.

The American novelist William Burroughs who, by his own account, was about as hopeless a case of addiction as could be imagined,[48] was cured by the use of apomorphine, a substance, which according to Burroughs, acts as a metabolic regulator counteracting the physiological changes that continued opiate use causes in the body. Apomorphine treatment differs from methadone maintenance in that it can be discontinued after it has taken effect.[49]

Both these treatments, however, fail to deal with the social and psychological bases of addiction. It may be that in many cases the use of a chemical blocking agent may in itself be sufficient. But if a truly open-minded approach is adopted it must not reject *a priori* the possibility that good medical practice may not always mean the withdrawal of the addict from his drug. The concept that the only legitimate goal of treatment is to suppress addiction is a *political* statement, elaborated over a number of years by legislative bodies. It may be that in the end medical science will arrive at the same conclusion, but it is essential that, whatever conclusion is reached, research ought not to be straightjacketed by preconceived moral judgments.

The British writer Peter Laurie has suggested, with some support from the eminent authority on schizophrenia, Dr. R. D. Laing, that the type of personality exhibited by young addicts before they have become addicted has strong parallels to the type of personality exhibited by young pre-schizophrenics.[50] Chein and his associates in their extensive study of addicted New York delinquents also noted the association of incipient schizophrenia with heroin use.[51] If, as Laing suggests, schizophrenia is the result of the patient's attempt to evade deep feelings of anxiety by creating a false outer personality, which hides his own inner emptiness and lack of identity,[52] then it can be seen immediately that opiates, which reduce anxiety feelings, may constitute an alternative strategy on the part of the individual to cope with a very threatening situation. If such should prove to be the case then very serious questions must be asked about whether opiate addiction should always be considered wrong in itself. In such a situation could opiates not be viewed in the same way as insulin to a diabetic?

Charles Winick has suggested that long-term statistics on addicts indicate that addiction may be a self-limiting condition, with a 'maturing-out' process leading to a ten-year average cycle from the beginnings of opiate use to final abandonment.[53] The implication is that the personal problems causing the original use may have been resolved or perhaps eliminated during the addiction cycle. Winick's thesis is not accepted by everyone, although it does seem to have attracted considerable agreement, as well as further supportive evidence. Of course it should be pointed out that Winick's observation is only a statistical trend and does not account for all cases, but if it does hold, it thus goes a long way toward exploding the conventional law enforcement wisdom that "the only cured addict is a dead addict." And it clearly offers support to Laurie's suggestion that opiate use may sometimes be an attempt on the part of an incipient schizophrenic to prevent himself from slipping over the edge into real madness. If the addict quits his addiction at a time when his personality disorders have subsided, then medically supervised opiate administration may be ultimately preferable, both in social and in personal terms, to the possibility of overt schizophrenia, which will probably be far more damaging than addiction itself, and with perhaps less chance of recovery.

The relationship between addiction and schizophrenia is merely one example of the type of thing that ought to be fully, and fearlessly, investigated. It is only in this way that we will ever achieve substantive knowledge of just what drug addiction is all about. But in this search two conditions must be emphasized: (1) No prejudgments should be allowed, and addiction must be viewed in complete separation both from the law and from existing social judgments; thus the a *priori* assumption that the only legitimate goal of drug treatment can be the elimination of drug use must be rejected; (2) there need not be one *best* way of treating addiction, but rather many ways, each of which may have special relevance to particular individuals.

Both these conditions imply some changes in the law. We will return to this in the last chapter, with specific proposals. Apart from specific legal arrangements, it is obvious that a changed public climate is necessary also, a climate in which the addict is viewed not with revulsion or self-righteousness, but with compassion and sympathy. This point is best illustrated by two quotations, the first by a lawyer, the second by a team of social science researchers.

Nowhere is there found among the advocates of criminal sanction an expression of concern for anything but freeing society from the depredations of drug sellers and drug users. Concern over the causes of addiction and the plight of the addict find very little place in the criminal sanction approach. So long as the chief concern is 'getting the addict off the street' and sending the peddlars to prison for long terms, the sky is the limit on what may be expected in the way of penalties.[54]

The addict is not simply an alien specimen that can be placed under a microscope, coldly dissected, or otherwise displayed to our disinterested and detached observation. He is a human being; that, in itself, is enough to implicate us. No matter how offensive or destructive we may find his behavior, we cannot regard him as a merely noxious object, an insensate thing, or less than human without to some degree dehumanizing ourselves. . . . He is one of us. His character and actions have consequences for us, as ours do for him. As members of a common society, we share in the responsibility for the conditions that have helped make him what he is, insofar as these conditions are subject to human control. . . . No matter how low he sinks, he cannot lose his right to justice; the lower he sinks, the greater is his claim to our concern.[55]

Footnotes

[1] Government of Canada. Department of National Health and Welfare. *Annual Reports* for years 1962 to 1968.

[2] Wolfgang Schmidt, "The Prevalence of Alcoholism and Drug Addiction in Canada," *Addictions*, vol. 15, no. 3 (Fall, 1968), p. 32.

[3] Alex Richman and Barry Humphrey, "Epidemiology of Criminal Narcotic Addiction in Canada," *Bulletin on Narcotics*, vol. 21, no. 1 (January-March, 1969), p. 33, Table III.

[4] House of Commons. *Debates* (June 7, 1961), p. 5983.

[5] George H. Stevenson, *op. cit.*

[6] Alcoholism and Drug Addiction Research Foundation of Ontario. *Seventeenth Annual Report*, (1967), p. 125, Table X.

[7] See, for example, Lady Frankau, "Canadian Narcotic Addicts in England — The Experience of One Physician," *Addictions*, vol. 11, no. 1, (Summer, 1964), p. 49.

[8] Richman and Humphrey, *op. cit.*, p. 37.

[9] 7-8 Edward VII, c. 50.

[10] House of Commons, *Debates* (1907-8), p. 12, 550.

[11] R. MacGregor Dawson, *William Lyon Mackenzie King: a Political Biography, 1874-1923* (Toronto, University of Toronto Press, 1958), p. 148.

[12] See, for instance, Lindesmith, *The Addict and The Law*, *op. cit.*, pp. 243-68, for a description of some of the methods that the Narcotics Bureau has employed to control all information about addiction that reaches the U.S. public, including the suppression of a Canadian film on drug addicts, produced by the National Film Board. See also Benjamin DeMott, "The Great Narcotics Muddle," *Harper's Magazine*, vol. 224, no. 1342 (March, 1962), pp. 46-54.

[13] House of Commons, *Debates* (1920), p. 1630.

[14] Emily Murphy, *The Black Candle* (Toronto, Thomas Allen, 1922).

[15] Byrne Hope Sanders, *Emily Murphy: Crusader* (Toronto, Macmillan, 1945), pp. 209-10.

[16] Murphy, *op. cit.*, p. 167.

[17] *Ibid.*, p. 288.

[18] Eldridge, *op. cit.*, p. 47.

[19] 9-10 Elizabeth II, c. 35. Part I ss. 3-6.

[20] *Op. cit.*, Part II, s. 17 (1).

[21] Austin M. Cooper, "Narcotics and the Burden of Proof: Offences under the Narcotic Control Act," *Addictions*, vol. 11, no. 1 (Summer, 1964), pp. 35-37. Cooper cites the case of R vs. Sharpe (1961) 131 C.C.C. 75.

[22] House of Commons, *Debates* (1961) pp. 5938-58 and 6218-19.

[23] 9-10 Elizabeth II, c. 35. Part I, s. 10 (3).

[24] *Op. cit.*, s. 10 (1) (c).

[25] *Op. cit.*, s. 10 (4).

[26] *Op. cit.*, s. 10 (9).

[27] R. St.J. Macdonald, "Narcotics, Addicts and the Law," *Addictions*, vol. 11, no. 1 (Summer, 1964), pp. 25-26.

[28] Eldridge, *op. cit.*, p. 33.

[29]Charles Winick, "Narcotics Addiction and its Treatment," *Law and Contemporary Problems*, vol. 22, no. 1 (Winter, 1957), pp. 31-32.

[30]See, for example, Dennis Aronowitz, "Civil Commitment of Addicts," *Columbia Law Review*, vol. 67, no. 3 (March, 1967), p. 407.

[31]Judge Morris Ploscowe, "Some basic problems in drug addiction and suggestions for research," in Joint Committee of the American Bar Association and the American Medical Association on Narcotics Drugs, Interim and Final Reports; *Drug Addiction: Crime or Disease?* (Bloomington, Indiana, Indiana University Press, 1961).

[32]Chein, *op. cit.*, pp. 22-23. See also "The varieties of drug experience," *Transaction*, vol. 5, no. 10 (October, 1968), p. 5, citing a study by Jordan Scher.

[33]John D. Harris, *The Junkie Priest: Father Daniel Egan, S.A.* (New York, Pocket Books, Inc., 1965), pp. 111-24.

[34]Aronowitz, *op. cit.*, p. 410.

[35]Macdonald, op. cit., p. 30.

[36]See, for example, Erving Goffman, *Asylums: Essays on the Social Situation of Mental Patients and other Inmates* (Garden City, N.Y., Anchor, 1961) and Thomas Szasz, *Law, Liberty, and Psychiatry* (New York, Macmillan, 1963).

[37]J. D. Armstrong and R. E. Turner, "Special Problem Groups: alcoholics, drug addicts, sex offenders," in W. T. McGrath, ed., *Crime and its Treatment in Canada* (Toronto, Macmillan, 1965), p. 443.

[38]Lewis Yablonsky, *Synanon: The Tunnel Back* (Baltimore, Penguin Books, 1967) provides a thoroughly detailed and entirely sympathetic study of Synanon.

[39]A highly critical look at Synanon is provided by Peter Collier, "The House of Synanon," *Ramparts*, vol. 6, no. 3 (October, 1967), pp. 48-54.

[40]Joseph Shelly and Alexander Bassin, "Daytop Lodge — a New Treatment Approach for Drug Addicts," *Corrective Psychiatry and Journal of Social Therapy*, vol. 11, no. 4 (July, 1965).

[41]Joe Pilati, "Schism on 14th Street: The Daytop explosion," *The Village Voice*, vol. 14, no. 6 (Nov. 21, 1968).

[42]John A. O'Donnell, "The rise and decline of a subculture," *Social Problems*, vol. 15, no. 1 (Summer, 1964), p. 84.

[43]Lady Frankau, *op. cit.*

[44]Eldridge, *op. cit.*, pp. 116-17.

[45]Quoted in Edwin M. Schur, *Crimes Without Victims: Deviant Behavior and Public Policy* (Englewood Clifts, N.J., Prentice-Hall, 1965), p. 152.

[46]The black writer Claude Brown has described the 'plague' of heroin addiction that swept through Harlem in the 1950s, and how this plague was slowed down, neither by law enforcement nor by medical treatment, but by the arrival on the Harlem scene of the militant Black Muslim movement. "In a way, it was a good thing that the Muslim faith was gaining ground in Harlem, because it gave something to the junkies. . . . When a junkie came out of jail or when he came back from getting a cure, it was the rule to just come back on the streets and do the same things he had been doing all along. Now it was different. . . . Now the junkies had a place to go, those who could accept the teachings of the Muslims. . . . It gave them a sense of being somebody, a sense of importance. All the time before they became Muslims, I suppose there was a feeling of insignificance that led them to self-destruction in one form

or another. It was just not being anybody. Now they were somebody, a part of something. I suppose that's all they needed." Claude Brown, *Manchild in the Promised Land* (New York, Macmillan, 1965), pp. 331-32.

[47]Eldridge, *op. cit.*, pp. 157-60. *Harper's Magazine*, vol. 237, no. 1422 (November, 1968), p. 145.

[48]"I had not taken a bath in a year nor changed my clothes or removed them except to stick a needle every hour in the fibrous grey wooden flesh of terminal addiction. . . . I could look at the end of my shoe for eight hours. I was only roused to action when the hourglass of junk ran out." William S. Burroughs, "Deposition: a Testimony Concerning a Sickness," in *Naked Lunch* (New York, Grove Press, 1966), p. xli.

[49]William S. Burroughs, "Kicking Drugs," *Harper's Magazine*, vol. 235, no. 1406 (July, 1964).

[50]Peter Laurie, *Drugs: Medical, Psychological, and Social Facts* (Harmondsworth, Middlesex, Penguin Books, 1967), pp. 140-42.

[51]Chein *et al, op. cit.*

[52]R. D. Laing, *The Divided Self* (Harmondsworth, Middlesex, Penguin Books, 1965).

[53]Charles Winick, "Maturing-out of Narcotic Addiction," *Bulletin on Narcotics*, vol. 14, no. 7 (Jan.-March 1962).

[54]Eldridge, *op. cit.*, pp. 105-6.

[55]Chein *et al, op. cit.*, pp. 3-4 and 326.

The Great Marijuana Scare

4

"Much of the irrational juvenile violence and killing that has written a new chapter of shame and tragedy is traceable directly to this hemp intoxication."[1] So wrote Mr. Harry Anslinger, for many years the guiding spirit of the U.S. Narcotics Bureau, and a man perhaps more responsible than anyone else in the world for the great marijuana scare that presently bedevils legislators, agitates educational authorities, and fills our jails and prisons with thousands of young people. I use the phrase 'the great marijuana scare' advisedly for there can be no doubt that, whatever final conclusions one draws, much of what has been publicly said and written about the subject, especially on the official level, has been garish and baseless fantasy. For many years the scare tactics of the U.S. Narcotics Bureau and of those who parrotted them in other countries went largely unanswered. Now, however, there has arisen at the other end of the spectrum an equivalent threat to good sense, this time emanating from the hippie philosophers of the 'pot will save the world' school. Anyone who wishes to make an honest effort to get at the truth behind the marijuana scare will have to pick their way between the Scylla and Charybdis of this emotional debate.

'Marijuana' – or 'Marihuana', the spelling is optional – is the Spanish-derived name commonly applied in North America to *Cannabis Sativa L* – the technical name for the hemp plant that grows freely all over the world. Cannabis is dioecious, that is, it has separate male and female plants as part of its reproductive process. Resin and its components in the flowering tops of the female plant provide the well-known hallucinogenic effects. The plant has, however, a number of other uses, of which the manufacture of rope, and the production of an oil used in paints and varnishes are among the more prominent. In North America, what is commonly sold as marijuana is a collection of dried flowers and leaves, seeds, and miscellaneous other parts of the plant (along with assorted impurities often introduced under the name of marijuana, but including anything from oregano and green tea, to catnip). To its devotees, the most prized part of the marijuana plant is the sticky brown resin that accumulates at the end of a marijuana cigarette when smoked. Cannabis resin is known in North America as *hashish* – a term of Arabic origin – and is sometimes imported directly from the Middle East and sold in the form of compressed cubes wrapped in tinfoil. Hashish appears to be a much more potent drug than the milder marijuana found in North America. Some have used the comparison of whisky to beer, although connoisseurs are more apt to refer to the difference between a fine vintage wine and a bottle of cheap *vin ordinaire*. The chemically active agent in cannabis, tetrahydrocannabinol (THC) has now been synthesized in the laboratory. There have been claims that THC has even made an appearance on the illegal market. Although this fact has yet to be proved, such a development would be of great importance for law enforcement authorities, for the attractiveness of marijuana and hashish as a target for police investigation has always been that it is bulky, easily identifiable by sight, and has a very strong and unmistakeable odor when smoked. Although marijuana can be eaten or even drunk as a tea, smoking seems to be the almost universal form of use in North America. Now that the THC has been synthesized, however, the same effects can possibly be brought about by the simple swallowing of an odorless pill.

Although the great marijuana scare is a rather recent public commotion in North America – beginning in the later 1930s under the orchestration of the U.S. Narcotics Bureau, dying down in the next twenty-five years, and then rising up out of all proportion in the second half of the 1960s – nevertheless the cannabis 'problem' has in fact been with us for the last five thousand years, and probably longer. It was mentioned in the writings of Chinese Emperor Shen Nung,[2] who was something of a pioneer pharmacologist, in 2737 B.C., although it must have been well-known long before then. Many Chinese did not like the drug very much; their suspicions about its effects may be seen in the description they applied to it – 'Liberator of Sin'. Some, however, called it the 'Delight Giver'. At some point in the first millennium B.C. cannabis use was introduced into India and found a much more responsive market.³ Cannabis does not appear to have any wide popularity in China in the twentieth century, but through the centuries since its introduction, it has remained an important part of life in India. The equivalent of our North American marijuana is called *bhang* in India and is considered a very crude and cheap product. *Ganja* is a more refined form of marijuana, which is widely used and appreciated for its quality. *Charas* is the Indian name applied to cannabis resin and has the reputation of being one of the most potent forms of cannabis to be found anywhere.

There is evidence of the presence of cannabis in Europe as early as the fifth century B.C.,⁴ although the use of hemp for rope-making was introduced later. Its use seems to have largely disappeared, however, only to be reintroduced by contact with the Islamic culture of the Middle East. After Marco Polo had travelled to the East in the thirteenth century he related to his Western audience the strange story of the Assassins led by the Old Man of the Mountain. Young men, it seemed, were being given a drug, and after falling asleep were transported to a beautiful garden that the Old Man of the Mountain had specially grown on a mountain in the midst of the desert. Here they awoke to a dream-like world of flowers and music and beautiful maidens. They believed themselves to be in Paradise, but after a time the Old Man would put them once more to sleep and have them brought into his presence, whereupon they would be told that they must accomplish a certain mission, usually an assassination, if they wished to return to the magic garden of delights. In this way the Old Man built up a fanatical band of terrorists who furthered his power and dominion over a wide area.⁵ The association of the name *assassin* with hashish led to the notion that hashish had played a major part in this remarkable story. One popular view is that the murderous fanaticism of the terrorists was caused directly by the hashish – this is an argument often dredged up to substantiate the alleged association of marijuana with violent behavior – but in another variant the hashish is seen as part of the celestial pleasures the Old Man set out as incentives to his Assassins. In a recent study the eminent Islamic scholar Bernard Lewis has suggested that association of hashish with the sect is "almost certainly untrue". Contrary to the view that the word *assassin* derives from the word *hashish*, Lewis suggests that "in all probability it was the name that gave rise to the story, rather than the reverse".[6] Thus the familiar spectre of the bloodthirsty Assassins 'hopped-up' on hashish so often invoked by the fear-mongers may be just another myth.

The first real reintroduction of cannabis to Europe came in the nineteenth century when a group of Parisian intellectuals, of which the most prominent were Charles Baudelaire and Théophile Gauthier, formed a society, called *Le Club des Hachichins*, where they smoked charas, or Indian hashish, as part of wild and uninhibited debauches. Unlike less articulate users they were not content to simply enjoy themselves in private but instead suffered from the writers' urge to tell all. Baudelaire in *Les Paradis Artificiels* and Gauthier in *Le Hachich* and *Le Club des Hachichins* recounted lurid and exotic tales of the drug's effects, thus creating much of the same public reaction of mingled fascination and moral outrage as had greeted De Quincey's *Confessions of an English Opium-Eater*, which both Baudelaire and Gauthier greatly admired. As with all such works, one never knows where the drug's effects stop and the already fertile imagination of the artist begins. Gauthier described the joys of hashish in a manner that undoubtedly shocked and fascinated the more conventional Parisians.

I was in that blessed state of hashish that the Orientals call *kief*. I was no longer aware of my body; the connection between matter and spirit was slender; I moved by my own will in a milieu which offered no resistance.

It is in this way, I imagine, that spirits must act in the fragrant world in which we travel after death.

A bluish mist, an Elysian day, a reflection of an azure grotto, formed in the room an atmosphere in which I could see wavering shapes vaguely tremble. This atmosphere, at the same time fresh and tepid, humid and perfumed, enveloped me like bath water in its enervating gentleness; if I wished to change my place, the caressing air made a thousand voluptuous ripples around me; a delicious languor took possession of my senses and returned me to the sofa where I subsided like a discarded garment.

I understood then the pleasure which, following their degrees of perfection, spirits and angels feel when crossing the ethers and the heavens, and how eternity must be spent in Paradise.

Nothing material mingled with this ecstasy; no terrestrial desire altered its purity. Indeed, love itself could add nothing to it, and a hashishist Romeo would have forgotten Juliette. The poor girl, leaning among the jasmins, would have extended in vain her beautiful arms of alabaster from the top of the balcony across the night. Romeo would have remained at the bottom of the silken ladder and, even though I am desperately in love with the angel of youth and the beauty created by Shakespeare, I must confess that the most beautiful girl of Verona, for a hashishist, is not worth the trouble of disturbing oneself.

Moreover, although charmed to be sure, I regarded with complacency the garland of ideally beautiful women who crowned the fresco with their divine nudity. I watched the gleam of their satin shoulders, the sparkling of their silvery bosoms, their rosy-soled feet, their opulent, undulating hips, without the slightest sense of temptation. The seductive spectres which troubled St. Anthony held no power over me.[7]

Anything that promised pleasures greater than sex was bound to provoke interest. Baudelaire spoke of hashish-taking as part of *le goût de l'Infini* – "the taste for the infinite" – and maintained that the final state of the hashish smoker was to believe himself to have become of God. "... All these things were created *for me, for me, for me!* For me humanity laboured, was martyred, burned – to provide the pasture, the *pabulum* for my implacable appetite for emotion, knowledge, and beauty!"[8] But Baudelaire was not completely sold on the idea of hashish. Some believed that the drug could be made into a productive instrument for enhancing the powers of human thought – thus antedating current hippie philosophizing by over a century. Baudelaire denied this point, however, and in terms just as relevant today as then.

... hashish reveals nothing to the individual except himself. It is true that the individual is, in a sense, multiplied to the third power and pushed to the extreme, and it is equally certain that these impressions survive the orgy. ... But I beg them to consider that the thoughts, upon which they count to such a great degree, are not in truth so beautiful as they appeared under their momentary disguise, overlaid with magic tinsel. They hold more of the earth than of heaven in them, and owe a great deal of their beauty to the nervous agitation and avidity with which the mind casts itself upon them. This hope is therefore a vicious circle: even if we admit for the moment that hashish gives, or at least enhances, genius, they forget that it is of the nature of hashish to diminish the free will, and what it gives with one hand it thus takes with the other, that is to say, it gives imagination without the means of profiting by it.[9]

In the 1850s an American writer, Bayard Taylor, introduced the idea of hashish-eating to North America with an account of his personal experiences with the drug in Damascus. Another anonymous American described his five-year enslavement to the drug in the same city. These reports perhaps prompted a young American, Fitzhugh Ludlow, to do his own experimentation, which was later written up with lavish detail, and not a little literary distinction, in *The Hasheesh Eater*.[10]

These experiments by French and American *literati* did not cause a great rise in popular consumption of hashish. Perhaps the exotic Oriental trappings frightened more people than they attracted. Certainly hashish use never even began to threaten the popularity of alcohol in the Western world. In the twentieth century cannabis became a part of North American life in the form of the much less potent marijuana as used by Mexican-Americans who imported the habit from Mexico. From this group marijuana use spread to other poor and disadvantaged groups such as the ghetto blacks and the urban poor. In the 1920s little public concern was expressed about the practice, and only a few American states passed laws against it. Then in 1937 the great marijuana scare arose. From research done into the period it seems incontestable that it was the U.S. Narcotics Bureau that was behind the sudden flare-up of public concern where there had been none before. Although only a few years earlier the Bureau had expressed no particular worry about the use of marijuana, it suddenly discovered in the late 1930s that the hemp plant was the 'assassin of youth',[11] and, using its commanding position as repository of supposedly authoritative information, directed a widespread publicity campaign against the horrors of the drug, inspiring a spate of atrocity-laden stories in the press and agitating both Congressional and state legislators into a froth over stopping this newly discovered menace. The reason for the Bureau's sudden concern is not hard to find. In the depression years and with the opiate problem diminishing from its high point in the 1920s, the Bureau found that its annual appropriations from Congress were declining. One obvious answer to this bureaucratic crisis was to create a new drug menace to justify the Bureau's continued existence. With the Bureau's command over information and communications in the narcotics field this did not prove to be a very difficult task.[12] Such behavior on the part of a government agency need not shock us too much. As William Burroughs remarks in his novel *Naked Lunch*, "Bureaus cannot live without a host, being true parasitic organisms."[13] This is particularly true of agencies that deal with so-called 'deviant' behavior, whether social or political. Since the successful elimination of the behavior in question would lead to the dissolution of the agency, there is usually a certain ambivalence on the agency's part. Thus it has been seriously suggested that in the depths of the Cold War in the 1950s the FBI actually kept the decayed and cadaverous U.S. Communist party alive through the financial contributions and participation of undercover FBI agents.

Today, as we shall see later, the most prominent arguments used by the opponents of liberalizing the legal status of marijuana, including the Narcotics Bureau, is the alleged connection between marijuana and heroin. It is very interesting, then, that in 1937 the Bureau not only failed to emphasize this point but in fact denied it. A Congressman questioning Mr. Anslinger inquired if "the marihuana addict graduates into a heroin, an opium or a cocaine user?" Mr. Anslinger replied directly: "No, sir; I have not heard of a case of that kind. I think it is an entirely different class. The marihuana addict does not go in that direction."[14] Instead the Bureau emphasized the connection between marijuana and crimes of violence. Rape and murder, moral degeneracy and debauchery, insanity and death, all lurked within the weed. And moreover, just as prohibitionists are convinced that a single sip of the Demon Rum will make a person into a hopeless life-long drunkard, so too the moralistic fanatics of the Narcotics Bureau were at pains to make it known that a single puff of the noxious plant would mean an immediate decline into the depths of depravity. The result was the passage of the *Marihuana Tax Act* of 1937, a bizarre piece of legislation that states that to grow or have possession of marijuana one must pay the U.S. Treasury Department for a tax stamp, which is never provided. Robert de Ropp, a biochemist and a writer generally modest in his opinions, has declared the Act to be a "semi-imbecile piece of legislation" and "a barbed-wire entanglement of prohibitive legislation that has been erected around this harmless weed by various busybodies who take a professional pride in curtailing the liberties of their fellow-men."[15] Others have been even less charitable than Dr. de Ropp.

It is not our task here to evaluate American legislation at any length. The passage of the *Marihuana Tax Act* does provide, however, a dramatic demonstration of some of the forces at work behind the prohibition of marijuana. The history of Canadian legislation is less clear-cut in its outlines than the American. As with the outlawing of opiates, Canada moved against marijuana much sooner than the United States, but did not indulge in some of the excesses of the American experience.

Possession or sale of cannabis became a serious offence in Canada in the early 1920s, when by Order in Council "cannabis indica (Indian Hemp) or Hasheesh, or its preparations or compounds or derivatives, or their preparations or compounds" were added to the schedule of outlawed drugs in the *Opium and Narcotic Drug Act*.[16] Judge Emily Murphy, in her 1922 book *The Black Candle*, had maintained that marijuana was a new menace that caused addiction, insanity, and death, although she also noted that its use was "as yet" comparatively unknown in Canada.[17] There seems to be no indication on the part of the Government concerning the reasons for its action. Certainly no opposition Members were going to concern themselves with some weird alien herb probably used only by disreputable foreign dope fiends, and the Government did not bother to explain such a non-controversial action. And thus it was, amid an utter silence, that the parliamentary system launched us on a course that today sends thousands of young people to jail, and disrupts the entire legal system. Little did they know, in those far-off days, what they had wrought. By attaching cannabis to the narcotics law, they were attaching it to a piece of legislation whose penalties and enforcement powers were to escalate steadily over the next decades. Like a small marking on the side of a balloon, the cannabis provision expanded as the whole balloon expanded, until eventually it became distorted and grotesque. In point of fact, it never had the slightest reason for being there in the first place, since, as we shall see, there is no basis for cannabis to be linked pharmacologically, psychologically, sociologically, or just plain logically to the opiates in the same piece of legislation. Even the Americans passed a *separate* marijuana act.

In 1932 the *Opium and Narcotic Drug Act* was amended to allow retail druggists to sell or distribute preparations and remedies that contained no more than two grains of "soft extract of Cannabis sativa or its equivalent, in one fluid ounce, or, of a solid or semi-solid preparation, in one avoirdupois ounce. . . ."[18] This provision was repealed in 1946,[19] but its implementation in 1932 reveals two interesting points. It would seem that cannabis was used to some extent as a medicinal substance at the time and, second, there was no real concern in the early 1930s over the 'marijuana menace'. The

Government of the time simply said that they had received representations from druggists and that they had no objections to these suggestions.

In 1938, however, Parliament discussed cannabis problems in quite a different spirit. It may well be doubted that cannabis use had suddenly increased or that its problems had become any more acute. The Minister of Pensions and National Health, Mr. C. G. "Chubby" Powers, told the House of Commons that up to 1932 there had been only twenty-eight convictions for possession of cannabis.[20] Since he neglected to mention any figures for the following five years, they were probably not too startling. What had happened, however, to rouse Parliament's concern was the great marijuana scare in the United States. The previous year the Narcotics Bureau had rammed the *Marihuana Tax Act* through Congress and while Canada might be proud of the fact that she had moved against the incipient menace years previously, it might also seem that some more positive act would be appropriate to show that we were no slackers compared to the U.S. zealots. Accordingly the Government introduced an amendment to the *Opium and Narcotic Drug Act*, which made unauthorized cultivation of the hemp plant a criminal offence, subject on indictment to from six months to seven years imprisonment *and* a fine of from $200 to $1,000. The minimum sentence was mandatory, which is to say that if a defendant were convicted, at least six months and $200 would be imposed. The judge was to retain some flexibility in sentencing, however: "at the discretion of the judge," a violator could be whipped.[21] Mr. Powers, in introducing this rather extraordinary piece of legislation – as hemp grows wild all over the world, the law's intent was somewhat quixotic – reported the usual lurid stories of American origin, brought in the old story of the Assassins, referred to the drug as "habit forming," and maintained that it was sold largely to youth. At one point Mr. Powers stated that while it was a "new menace to the youth of the country" it could not be called a new drug since it had been known since the days of Homer. "Is that," former Prime Minister R. B. Bennett interjected brightly, "the reason Homer nodded?" To which Mr. Powers replied, "No, on the contrary, the effect is not to make people nod; it is exceedingly stimulating. It is probably the reason why there was an attack on Troy."[22] So much for all the learned theories on the causes of the Trojan war! Another member, quoting the eminent American cannabis authority, Mr. Harry J. Anslinger, solemnly exorcised this "assassin of youth – one of the greatest menaces which has ever struck that country."[23] Needless to say, such leaden-witted oratory did little to throw any enlightenment on a subject that to most Canadians was a perplexing and unknown quantity. If Parliament has, as some political scientists like to maintain, a leading role in educating public opinion, it certainly was not fulfilled at this time – if indeed, when one looks back over the whole rather sorry history of legislative blustering and blundering on the cannabis question, it was ever fulfilled.

The following year World War II began and the attention of Parliament turned to other and more important matters. The great marijuana scare quickly faded from political consideration. It was not until the mid-1960s that it arose again, and this time in a far more pervasive form than ever before. We will return later to the current controversy, but first we should take a searching look at just what this drug cannabis is, and what it does.

It is in a way unfortunate that the poetic effusions of Baudelaire, Gauthier, Ludlow, and of such contemporaries as Allen Ginsberg should be taken as universally applicable statements of what the cannabis experience is like. First of all, these are all persons with great literary and imaginative gifts. If you put a painting or a piece of music before persons who have already cultivated a sense of aesthetic appreciation you are apt to evoke a far more complex and suggestive reaction than if you present the same work to someone who pays little attention to such matters. The latter may well react, and may even be more deeply moved than those whose minds are already filled with preconceived categories – but in any event the reaction will likely be *different* from the reaction of the artist, and will almost certainly be less easily communicable to others than that of the artist who is more practiced in this activity. The cannabis experience may not mean the same thing to the less articulate as it does to the person whose fertile imagination lies close to the surface and is easily awakened. For example, Baudelaire also derived poetic ecstasies from the use of wine – yet we know enough about alcohol to laugh at any suggestion that it is fundamentally an aid to the free poetic imagination. It may be such as aid; but then again it may have nothing whatever to do with creativity. Yet imagine for a moment that we live in a society where cannabis is acceptable but alcohol forbidden. In such a situation it would most likely be the daring *avant-garde* artists who would dabble in the unlawful drug and write ecstatic accounts of their experiences. A curious public, wishing to know what alcohol was, would then be treated to magnificent flights of inspired fancy, and might be led into believing that it was alcohol itself that imparted such imaginative delights. Meanwhile many others, of less literary bent, might be drinking alcohol and doing nothing more than picking fights, vomiting or sinking into a stupor. This is put forward as a warning to those who would put too much stock in what poets and writers say about cannabis. They are, after all, a most unrepresentative sample.

Nor can individual statements by isolated persons be easily generalized into a theory. Anyone who sets out to inquire into the nature of the cannabis experience by questioning individuals on their subjective reactions will quickly find the task to be frustrating. Some say the drug produces complex hallucinations; others see no hallucinations whatever. Some find their perceptual awareness deepened; others fall asleep. Some claim that it changed their whole perspective on life; others that it meant nothing.

Scientific examinations based on a wider population offer a potentially more fruitful approach to the subject, but few substantive conclusions have been reached. The illegality and ill-repute of cannabis is undoubtedly the reason for this gap. In fact in both Canada and the United States it has been very difficult to carry out research into cannabis since in both countries the federal governments have been very loath to allow such work, not to speak of the attitude of the public. The reasoning seems to have been as follows: (a) we know that cannabis use is wrong, because it is illegal; (b) why waste time and valuable resources on research into a drug that already we have decided has no medical value? (c) if the research attempts to show that cannabis is not as bad as we have declared it to be, then we do not want such research anyway. If all this sounds suspiciously like "I know my prejudices, don't confuse me with facts," the resemblance is not co-incidental. In fact a professor at the University of Victoria in British Columbia who wanted to undertake a study of marijuana was refused permission by the Federal government on the grounds that any such study would be "valueless". The result of this type of attitude has been, not surprisingly, a lack of basic research on the subject.

The first important inquiry into the use of cannabis was also the most voluminous. In 1894 the British imperial government in India published in seven volumes of over 3,000 pages the results of a two-year study into the widespread use of cannabis among the Indian masses. The Indian Hemp Drug Commission, as it was called, carried out extensive interviews among a multitude of Indians from all walks of life. It concluded that:

1. There is no evidence of any weight regarding mental and moral injuries from the moderate use of these drugs.
2. Large numbers of practitioners of long experience have seen no evidence of any connection between the moderate use of hemp drugs and disease.
3. Moderation does not lead to excess in hemp any more than it does in alcohol. Regular, moderate use of ganja or bhang produces the same effects as moderate and regular doses of whiskey. Excess is confined to the idle and dissipated.[24]

This massive study was notable both for its fair-mindedness and for its comprehensiveness. Norman Taylor goes so far as to suggest that it will "probably always be the classic work on hemp."[25] The fact that it was carried out under the auspices of the British government at the zenith of the Victorian era makes its generous and tolerant conclusions doubly significant. They evidently agreed with the Indian writer who had suggested that

To forbid or even seriously to restrict the use of so holy and gracious an herb as the hemp would cause widespread suffering and annoyance. . . . It would rob the people of a solace in discomfort, of a cure in sickness, of a guardian whose gracious protection saves them from the attacks of evil influences. . . . So grand a result, so tiny a sin![26]

After the great marijuana scare in the late 1930s in the United States had given rise to a spate of cannabis atrocity stories, there were nevertheless some more moderate voices who suggested milder conclusions. This was, it must be remembered, a time when a newspaper like the Communist *New York Daily Worker* could straightforwardly print the following type of horror story.

Smoking of the weed is habit-forming. It destroys the will-power, releases restraints, and promotes insane reactions. Continued use causes the face to become bloated, the eyes bloodshot, the limbs weak and trembling, and the mind sinks into insanity. Robberies, thrill murders, sex crimes, and other offences result. . . .
The habit can be cured only by the most severe methods. The addict must be put into an institution, where the drug is gradually withdrawn,

his general health is built up, and he is kept there until he has enough will-power to withstand the temptation to again take to the weed.[27]

Dr. Robert P. Walton, who was a Professor of Pharmacology at the University of Mississippi, wrote a book in 1938 that viewed cannabis as being very dangerous indeed and even carried a commendatory blurb by Mr. Anslinger on the dust jacket. Yet Dr. Walton's book was in a very different class from the rantings of the Narcotics Bureau, and indeed he expressed fears that the punitive legislation embodied in the *Marihuana Tax Act* of the previous year – which he hoped would wipe out illicit use – might serve to eradicate legitimate research into the drug.[28] His fears, of course, proved only too correct.

There were two voices that arose in opposition to the official position of the federal government at this time, and that carried some weight with the general public – one voice from the U.S. Army and the other from an official investigation sponsored by the government of New York City. In 1925 a committee was appointed to investigate the use of cannabis by American soldiers stationed in the Panama Canal Zone. The committee found that the drug was not addictive and exercised no "appreciably deleterious influence" on the individual. In 1931 another such investigation revealed that "Delinquencies due to marijuana smoking which result in trial by military court are negligible in number when compared with delinquencies resulting from the use of alcoholic drinks which also may be classed as stimulants and intoxicants."[29] In a study that covered five hundred users for a one-year period, the investigation failed to turn up a single case of psychosis due to cannabis. Ten years later the editor of *The Military Surgeon* (the journal of the Association of Military Surgeons in the United States) declared that smoking cannabis was no more harmful than smoking tobacco, and termed the 1937 anti-cannabis legislation to be "ill-advised," "that it branded as a menace and a crime a matter of trivial importance."[30] In fairness it should be pointed out that two later studies of army users found evidence of a strong degree of habituation to the drug, although H. B. M. Murphy of McGill is critical of this finding on the grounds that the subjects' habituation may have been more toward their delinquent subculture, of which pot-smoking was a symbol, than to the drug itself.[31]

Far most important than these Army studies was the work of the LaGuardia Committee in New York. Faced with press hysteria about the cannabis 'menace', New York's colorful Mayor, Fiorello La-Guardia, acted in a manner quite uncharacteristic of politicians and decided that rather than buy cheap popularity by playing up massive arrests of the politically powerless cannabis users of Harlem, he would instead use the prestige of his office to sponsor a scientific inquiry into the drug to determine whether the great marijuana scare was in fact justified on rational grounds. Accordingly in 1938 he asked the New York Academy of Medicine to carry out a study of cannabis use. The Academy surveyed the existing literature and decided that a first-hand investigation was required, and in 1939 a Mayor's Committee on Marihuana was formed, composed of some leading New York medical officials. Sociological, clinical, and pharmacological studies were undertaken, with the full co-operation of the law-enforcement authorities in New York.

The sociological study was carried out in the Borough of Manhatten by six undercover police agents, who were ordered to make no arrests but simply to observe in detail the behavior of cannabis users. By these on-the-spot methods the following conclusions were reached.

... The cost of marihuana is low and therefore within the purchasing power of most persons.
The distribution and use of marihuana is centered in Harlem.
The majority of marihuana smokers are Negroes and Latin-Americans.
The consensus among marihuana smokers is that the use of the drug creates a definite feeling of adequacy.
The practice of smoking marihuana does not lead to addiction in the medical sense of the word.
The sale and distribution of marihuana is not under the control of any single organized group.
The use of marihuana does not lead to morphine or heroin or cocaine addiction and no effort is made to create a market for these narcotics by stimulating the practice of marihuana smoking.
Marihuana is not the determining factor in the commission of major crimes. ...
Juvenile delinquency is not associated with the practice of smoking marihuana.
The publicity concerning the catastrophic effects of marihuana smoking in New York City is unfounded.[32]

The clinical study was based on seventy-two prisoners drawn from New York penitentiaries, made up of sixty-five males and seven females, and including whites, Negroes, and Puerto Ricans.

Forty-eight of the group had smoked cannabis previously. When they were tested with the drug, it was found that a "mixture of euphoria and apprehension was generally present."[33] Much depended upon the circumstances in which the drug was taken whether general well-being or anxiety developed. No aggressiveness was observed of any kind, nor any form of erotic stimulation. When the subjects themselves controlled the dosage taken they voluntarily stopped well before acute intoxication set in. In three subjects, all with previous personality disorders, a "definite psychotic state" was brought about. "The conclusion seems warranted that given the potential personality make-up and the right time and environment, marihuana may bring on a true psychotic state."[34]

The effects of the drug on performance of psychomotor functions varied with the degree of complexity involved: simple functions were relatively unaffected, while more complex functions were considerably affected. Body steadiness and hand steadiness were most severely affected. Non-users were more affected in general than users. The ability to measure short periods of time and short linear distances was not measurably changed. There was no evidence that musical ability is improved by the use of cannabis.[35]

Testing of the effects of the drug on mental performance yielded the following results. The effects are only transitory. The degree of mental impairment is directly related to the dosage taken. Once again it was the most complex functions that were impaired the most, and the simplest the least. Non-users experience greater intellectual impairment for longer periods than users. The individual under cannabis tends to lose both speed and accuracy in mental functioning, but use of the drug does not appear to result in long-term mental deterioration.[36]

"Under the influence of marihuana the basic personality structure of the individual does not change but some of the more superficial aspects of his behavior show alteration." The drug increases feelings of relaxation, disinhibition, and self-confidence. The self-confidence tends to be expressed primarily in words rather than in aggressive activity. Disinhibition releases what is already latent in the individual's thoughts and emotions, but there are no reactions alien to his undrugged personality. Feelings of anxiety are also released. Inexpressive individuals who have difficulty in making social contacts are more prone to cannabis use than are more outgoing persons.[37]

Tests to determine attitudes toward family and community

found few marked changes between the drugged and undrugged states, although while only four out of fourteen subjects without cannabis said they would tolerate the public sale of the drug, eight were in favor after they had experience with cannabis. One significant difference was, however, that with the drug, subjects tended to tolerate more disorder in the organization of the community than when they were without the drug.[38] From the clinical study as a whole it was concluded that cannabis is not a drug of addiction, and that long-term users showed "no mental or physical deterioration which may be attributed to the drug."[39]

The LaGuardia Committee report is unique in North America in being the only large-scale overall study undertaken on the subject of cannabis with the full cooperation of a major government as well as its law enforcement agencies. The results of the study flatly contradicted the more grotesque fantasies proffered by the Narcotics Bureau, but they by no means constitute a *carte blanche* for free cannabis use. The clinical study clearly pointed out the personal dangers of cannabis use, especially in the release of anxiety feelings. There is also legitimate criticism to be directed at the methodology of the study: the size and selection of samples, the failure to provide control groups, the failure to provide placebo tests – that is, the use of harmless substitutes for cannabis without the subject's knowledge to determine how many of the drug's apparent effects are a result of the subject's expectations – and the failure to provide double-blind procedures in which the observer knows no more than the subject about the exact conditions of any given test (in order to eliminate the bias that the investigator's expectations impart to the subject's behavior). By contemporary social science standards, the LaGuardia report is methodologically defective; its conclusions must consequently be viewed with a certain reserve. But whatever its defects, it was infinitely better grounded in scientific fact than the opinions of many of its critics. In fact the net effect of the Panama Canal Zone and New York studies seems to have been to increase rather than to decrease the irrationality of those committed to uprooting the evil weed at all costs. The press was especially incensed as it was getting enormous mileage out of the marijuana menace.

There are a few other important studies of cannabis that were published about the same time as the LaGuardia Committee report; but after 1946 no major North American clinical studies were undertaken until very recently. The fact that the New York and

Panama studies had at least raised serious questions about the conventional wisdom should have led to a series of studies. But the legal and political status of cannabis seems to have made it forbidden fruit, not only to individuals but to scientists as well. This is inexcusable on any grounds. Despite the paucity of material and the admittedly tenuous nature of our knowledge we will now attempt to summarize what has been found since the LaGuardia report.

The first question that is probably troubling any reader who has never taken cannabis is just what the cannabis experience *is*. Although this is one of the most basic questions it is a difficult one to answer, for in a sense there are as many different cannabis experiences as there are cannabis users. There is, however, an old Persian tale that may help throw some light on the problem. It seems that there were three travellers who arrived at a city late at night after the gates had been closed. One of the travellers was a drinker of alcohol, one was an opium user, and one smoked hashish. The problem that confronted them was what to do now that the city gates were closed. The alcohol drinker, as was his wont, became belligerent and declared that they should smash the gates down and march in. The opium user lethargically announced that he was falling asleep and would simply rest there until the next morning. The hashish taker was contemptuous of both these attitudes and put forward what he thought to be a clever plan. "It's very simple," he confided with great profundity, "we'll go in through the keyhole!"

We know almost nothing about how cannabis works on the human mind in a chemical sense, but its effects certainly seem to be to *disorganize* to some degree the normal thought processes. It is not at all uncommon for pot smokers to get a series of 'brilliant' ideas while smoking and then to later realize that the ideas do not seem so brilliant in the cold light of sobriety. Hashish effects tend to resemble the hallucinogenic effects of LSD and mescaline across a wide range of phenomena (see Chapter 6 for a detailed examination of the hallucinogenic experience) but with the much less potent marijuana, the hallucinogenic effects are less pronounced.[40]

So far as observable behavior goes there is some degree of common agreement on the initial effects, which usually are: (a) dulling of attention; (b) talkative euphoria; (c) restlessness, excessive movement, and emotional instability; (d) possibly some distortion of the perception of space and time, depending on the dose; (e) lassitude and sleep if the dose is sufficient.[41] Euphoria can also be replaced by depression; mental activity can increase or decrease; the appetite is most likely to be sharpened, but is in some cases diminished; in some subjects awareness of their surroundings is enhanced, but in others drowsiness results. Experienced users are, however, much better able to regulate their intake so as to suppress unpleasant effects and to maximize the euphoric effects than are novice users. Repressed ideas are released but at the same time the work drive is reduced so that ideas are rarely embodied in actions.[42] There is a good deal of controversy over the alleged aphrodisiac effects of cannabis. Apparently in some persons sexual arousal as well as enjoyment is enhanced, although others report no particular sexual interests whatsoever during the use of the drug. We have already cited Gauthier's comment that the fairest maid of Verona could not tempt a hashish smoker. Perhaps a mild dosage of marijuana *could* be a sexual stimulant; but it could just as well as be a substitute for sexual desire.

The first major clinical study of cannabis effects since 1946 was conducted at the Boston University School of Medicine in 1968 despite "opposition from nearly every source". This study, conducted by Andrew Weil, Norman Zinberg, and Judith Nelsen, is the first attempt to study the effects of the type of marijuana used in North America in a controlled and neutral laboratory setting with double-blind procedures. Eight chronic student users were easily selected from the twenty-one to twenty-six age group, but the selection of marijuana-naive persons in the student population of Boston proved very difficult – nearly two months of interviewing were required to find a sufficient number of such persons, and those who were found seemed apologetic about the fact that they had not tried the drug! The situation thus revealed says much about the effectiveness of the present laws. Cigarettes were provided that contained strictly controlled dosages in three forms: (a) high-dose marijuana, with a small plug of tobacco at the end to mask the contents; (b) low-dose marijuana, with a greater amount of tobacco; (c) placebo cigarettes containing a mixture of the inactive male cannabis plant and tobacco. The marijuana used was of average North American strength. Dosages were administered in a double-blind fashion to the subjects who were then required to take certain tests. In this way neither the investigator nor the subject knew at the time whether the high dose, low dose or placebo was being smoked, thus reducing the factor of both the subject's and the investigator's expectations. The results of the experiment were as follows.

1. There were no adverse marijuana reactions. Observable effects were maximal at fifteen minutes after smoking, diminished between half an hour and an hour and were largely dissipated within three hours. No persistent effects were observed beyond this period. Nicotine reactions, however, were in some cases acute!

2. All chronic users became 'high' on a high dose of marijuana. Of the naive subjects, however, only one had an equivalent reaction – and he was the one naive subject who had expressed a desire to get 'high'.

3. There seemed to be consistently different reactions on the part of the two groups to identical doses.

4. Most subjects found high-dose cigarettes milder than either the low-dose or placebo cigarettes, which both contained tobacco. Most were able to distinguish marijuana from the placebo, but they all consistently tended to underrate the dosage of marijuana, indicating a mild subjective reaction to the drug.

5. Marijuana brought about an increase in heart-rate fifteen minutes after smoking, but this increase was statistically higher among chronic users than among the naive subjects.

6. Among naive subjects, there was no change in the respiratory rate after administration of marijuana; there was, however, a small increase in the rate of the chronic users, but one that was not clinically significant.

7. Despite widespread reports of dilated pupils, there was no change in pupil size.

8. Reddening of the eyes did take place and was directly related to the dosage. It was more prominent among the chronic users.

9. There was no significant change in blood-sugar levels. The sharp hunger displayed by marijuana smokers thus remains unexplained.

10. Effects of marijuana on continuous performance tests could not be detected for either group.

11. Testing of cognitive function showed gross impairment on the part of naive subjects after smoking, but chronic users started with good performance and improved slightly after marijuana use.

12. Testing to measure muscular coordination and attention showed impairment among naive subjects and improvement on the

part of chronic users – although the authors point out the probability that the latter may have become practiced in the test.

13. Marijuana did have an upward effect on the estimation of time, making events seem longer in duration than they were in reality.

14. Subjectively, the naive subjects reported few effects from the drug. Little euphoria, no perceptual distortions except of time, and no confusion resulted.

Some general conclusions were drawn from the study. The greater subjective effects experienced by the chronic users on the same dosage indicates a unique "reverse tolerance," that is, as use becomes more frequent, the amount needed to produce the required degree of intoxication *decreases*. This is in startling contrast to most other intoxicants. Another point was that with increasing experience with the drug, its effects are more easily suppressed. Moreover the chronic users expressed surprise over their effective performance on tests while 'high' – this surprise the authors found "remarkable," for "it is quite the opposite of the false sense of improvement subjects have under some psychoactive drugs that actually impair performance." Marijuana "appears to be a relatively mild intoxicant," when smoked in the form usually available in North America. It must be noted, however, that this conclusion applies only to marijuana, and not to hashish, nor to synthetic THC.[43]

It might be noted in passing that cannabis effects can be observed in animals as well as in humans. When monkeys were given THC, normal behavior patterns were disrupted and the animals showed clear signs of experiencing visual hallucinations – such as watching non-existent moving objects, or engaging in fights with imaginary antagonists. High dosages caused severe depressions, which in some instances led to death.[44] Complex behavior involving memory and visual discrimination was markedly disrupted.

Questions raised by the clinical studies are perplexing, and none more perplexing than the extreme differences exhibited by naive and experienced users. There are no widely accepted chemical or physiological explanations to account for this difference, although some hypotheses are now being tested by the Addiction Research Foundation of Ontario. We may also look elsewhere, to the social context in which cannabis is taken. It is now generally recognized that, especially in the case of hallucinogenic-type drugs, the drug itself may be less important than the *set* and the *setting*. The *set* refers to the expectations of the subject, and the *setting* to the environment in which the drug is taken. A study done in 1953 by Howard Becker – who is not only a leading sociologist but was also for a number of years a jazz pianist – emphasized particularly the *setting* as a factor. In terms that closely mesh with the clinical study of Weil and Zinberg, Becker found that naive users were unable to take marijuana for pleasure until they had been taught by more experienced users how to smoke it in an effective way, how to recognize the effects and connect them with the use of the drug, and how to enjoy the sensations derived from its use. Becoming a marijuana user is thus a *learning process* and, in Becker's view, individual motives may emerge only in the course of the experience itself and cannot always be ascribed to prior predispositions of the individual.[45] Certainly it is a common observation among those who have tried cannabis that the first attempt is almost always disappointing. Some in fact give it up immediately as they derive no enjoyment and perhaps some discomfort from the irritating smoke. Another interesting observation that confirms the Becker thesis is that among young people in North America pot-smoking is almost exclusively a social or communal event. Only the more chronic users are likely to smoke by themselves when no one else is available.

Since the great marijuana scare has been revived in the 1960s a number of conflicting points of view on the problem have been debated in the press and by the mass media. As this has involved a great deal of confusion, it would be useful to examine some of these controversies in the light of medical and scientific knowledge. First of all we might look at some of the arguments put forward by the opponents of cannabis use and the opponents of changes in the law, and then go on to examine some of the pro-cannabis viewpoints put forward by its proponents.

1. *Cannabis is a drug of addiction.* This used to be a common claim on the part of law enforcement authorities, but now that the subject has become a matter of serious debate, this argument in its pure form has been largely abandoned. Scarcely anyone would seriously claim any longer that cannabis is physically addictive in the sense that heroin or morphine are addictive, that is to say, that the withdrawal of the drug brings about a characteristic abstinence syndrome. Even in the East where the chronic cannabis user tends to consume an amount far in excess of the average North American user, withdrawal rarely brings about specific physiological symp-

toms, and these are quite mild compared to opiate withdrawal.[46] In North America, studies by Allentuck and Bowman in 1942[47] and Freedman and Rockmore in 1946[48] found no evidence of addiction to the North American variety of cannabis. The Presidential Commission on Law Enforcement in the United States recently backed up this finding.[49]

Some of the proponents of cannabis use think that they have dismissed the whole question of addiction if they can show that there is no analogy to the opiates. But why should we be so obsessed with the model of heroin addiction that we cannot recognize other types of habituation? In fact medical opinion has in recent years been shifting away from the drawing of strict lines between addictive/non-addictive drugs, and toward a more comprehensive definition of habituation, which would include psychic dependence on a substance even without the usual physiological withdrawal symptoms. It is quite evident that in Eastern countries there are many persons whose lives centre so closely around cannabis – especially of the potent hashish variety – that they are, for all practical purposes, 'addicted'. And even in North America, it is true, as Murphy states, that cannabis "does offer an escape from the world, and for individuals whose personal inadequacy or social misery are great enough the desire for such escape may lead to a rejection of life without the drug, which is indistinguishable from addiction."[50] On the other hand, we cannot assume that dependence is necessarily an evil that must be rooted out at all costs, since, as McGlothlin suggests, "many forms of acceptable behavior can be included under this category. *The assessment of the harmfulness of psychic dependence must be based on the consequences of the behavior rather than its existence.*"[51] What we must get away from is the notion that if a drug is physically addictive it is harmful and should be outlawed, but that if it is not physically addictive it is harmless and should not be outlawed. Problems of drug control are far more complex than this. But what we can say of cannabis is that while moderate or occasional use will not in itself create dependence, chronic indulgence may establish such a relationship. Having said this we ought also to point out that the same is true of alcohol, and it is at least possible that the pot-head will be more easily withdrawn from his dependence than the alcoholic from his.

2. *Cannabis use leads to heroin.* The RCMP state that seventy per cent of all heroin addicts started with cannabis. This is put for-

ward as 'proof' that cannabis *leads* to heroin use. In many ways this is a very curious type of argument, so curious that, as we noted earlier, even Mr. Anslinger failed to support such an argument in the 1930s. It has become much more common since, to the point where it seems to constitute the main pillar in the anti-cannabis edifice. As a pillar it is made of pretty weak stuff.

There are two ways the argument can be made. First of all it can rest on the simple statistical tendency of heroin addicts to have smoked marijuana before they became addicted.[52] Even on this basis it is obvious that people become addicted *without* ever using cannabis,[53] but the real criticism of this approach is a disrespectful "so what?" Why start with heroin and work backwards? Why not start with cannabis and go on from there? Although no one knows for sure the number of cannabis users in North America it is quite obvious that they vastly exceed the number of heroin users. No one has established a statistical correlation beginning with cannabis and leading to heroin. A highly respected authority on juvenile and adolescent problems has concluded that cannabis "only occasionally is followed by heroin usage, probably in those who would have become heroin addicts as readily without the marijuana."[54] An extensive study done in the Oakland, California slum areas among mainly Negro and Mexican juveniles recently found that marijuana users were quite distinct from the heroin users and were in fact quite contemptuous of the latter. As one pot-head described a heroin addict: "He's lame, he's a chump to get into that bag."[55] And, in any event, why choose cannabis as a causal factor in heroin addiction? No doubt more heroin addicts once drank alcohol, or even milk for that matter, than have used cannabis. One anti-marijuana crusader in the 1930s had the courage to take the marijuana-heroin argument to its logical conclusion. As he explained

Slowly, insidiously, for over three hundred years, Lady Nicotine was setting the stage for a grand climax. The long years of tobacco using were but an introduction and training for marijuana use. Tobacco, which was first smoked in a pipe, then as a cigar, and at last as a cigarette, demanded more and more of itself until its supposed pleasures palled, and some of the tobacco victims looked about for something stronger. Tobacco was no longer potent enough.[56]

The same writer quoted a gangster as saying: "Every cigarette smoker is a prospect for the dope ring via the marihuana road. Millions of boys and girls now smoke. Think of the unlimited new market!"[57]

Statistically speaking, one can show a lot of relationships that really have little *actual* validity. It could no doubt be shown that in urban areas almost all women who become pregnant have watched television before becoming pregnant. So television causes pregnancy? Sometimes the cannabis-heroin relationship is expressed so crudely that it is almost as ridiculous as the television-pregnancy relationship. Recently in Ontario a girl was convicted of selling heroin and the judge took the opportunity to assert that because the accused had a previous marijuana conviction, her case "disproved" the theory that marijuana does not lead to heroin![58]

Perhaps sensing the flimsiness of the statistical relationship argument, an alternative presentation is sometimes made on the basis that the 'kicks' that cannabis provides at first, diminish with subsequent use so that the user begins looking for new and more powerful thrills, at which point heroin enters the scene. There is not the slightest pharmacological or psychological basis for this theory. In fact, as the Weil-Zinberg study indicates clearly, the cannabis 'high', far from diminishing with continuous use, actually increases so that lower dosages can be used. But unless a firm link can be established between the pharmacological *effects* of cannabis and the use of heroin, the statistical argument is without meaning.

There is, however, one realistic basis for linking the two drugs. Both cannabis and heroin can only be obtained illegally. The cannabis user is perhaps put in contact with a subculture in which heroin is available, although this would have been much more likely a number of years ago than today, with widespread middle-class and 'hippie' cannabis use. But to use this as an argument for maintaining cannabis in its *illegal* status is to defy all logic. If we are afraid of heroin, the whole point is to get the cannabis users away from the addict subculture, not to force them into a closer relationship.

3. *Cannabis use leads to violence and crime.* This is the most venerable argument used by opponents of cannabis in North America; but although the oldest it is by no means the most respectable argument. In fact, even in the 1930s, when the Narcotics Bureau was widely disseminating stories of children butchered, mothers raped, and innocent bystanders hacked to death by marijuana-crazed lunatics running amok in decent middle-class streets, more scientific inquiry failed to substantiate such a tendency on a general scale. Two

substantial statistical studies conducted by Bromberg could find little correlation between crime and cannabis.[59] More recently Moraes Andrade analysed 120 cannabis users alleged to have committed crimes while under the influence of the drug and concluded that criminal activity would have taken place without the drug.[60] It is interesting that the ubiquitous Mr. Anslinger showed his dedication to the spirit of free inquiry by castigating the U.N. Commission on Narcotics for allowing a study such as that of Andrade to be published in a U.N. journal. Mr. Anslinger, who was a most powerful figure in the international organizations on narcotics, wanted no more articles that "run counter to the aims pursued by the Commission."[61] This is an example of just what rational inquiry in this area is up against. In fact, the intolerant authoritarianism not only betrays a case that is weak, but one that is scarcely credible. As Murphy sums up our existing knowledge: "Most serious observers agree that cannabis does not, per se, induce aggressive or criminal activities, and that the reduction of work drive leads to a negative correlation with criminality rather than a positive one."[62] The Blumer study among Oakland juveniles found that the pot-heads were the 'cool' types, not delinquent, and avoided trouble. The rowdies much preferred alcohol.[63] Finally, the U.S. Presidential Commission on Crime in 1967 failed to substantiate any clear relationship between cannabis and crime.[64]

Cannabis opponents often argue that the drug's use leads to sloth and lethargy. Clearly this point is not compatible with the violence and crime argument. In a sense the restriction of cannabis use in the past to marginal and ethnic groups, such a Mexicans and Negroes, as well as to urban slum areas may have led to confusion between the effects of poverty and discrimination and those of cannabis. There is also an element of class-bias involved, with judgments about the horrors of cannabis really being judgments about the moral quality of life among lower-class minority groups. The illegal status of the drug obviously contributes to its criminal reputation. All in all, the cannabis-crime connection very much resembles the opiates-crime connection that we have already discussed in a previous chapter. But whereas the opiate addict usually is a criminal inasmuch as he must steal to pay for his habit, the cannabis user generally lacks such compulsion. Finally, however, it must be said that cannabis is unpredictable and capricious in its effects: it is certainly possible that the odd individual might commit a crime or act of violence under its influence, and there can be no doubt that such cases have occurred. But in general its effects would seem to be in the other direction. By contrast, alcohol is well known, indeed notorious, for inducing belligerence and aggression. There is no doubt at all that a large number of crimes and acts of violence are committed under its influence.

4. *Cannabis is damaging to the mind and body.* In India it has been shown that excessive consumption of hashish leads to frequent occurrence of various ailments, such as conjunctivitis, chronic bronchitis, tuberculosis, and various digestive disorders. It must be understood, however, that Indian users tend to consume far more of the drug than the typical North American (both in terms of potency of dose and frequency of use). The users of *bhang*, which is more equivalent to North American marijuana, showed none of these distressing signs.[65] A study conducted among U.S. Army personnel in 1946 found no evidence of physical deterioration among some 300 men with an average history of seven years marijuana use.[66] Obviously over-indulgence in cannabis can bring physical harm to the individual, just as over-indulgence in almost anything will have bad effects. What is important, however, is that there is no evidence that moderate use of mild North American marijuana brings about debilitating physical consequences. Two warnings are, however, in order: hashish *may* be dangerous to the health, especially if used in large quantities; and we ought, after the revelations concerning tobacco and lung cancer, to be very suspicious about any substance drawn into the body regularly over a long period, especially by smoking. We cannot say that cannabis has been *proved* to be harmless; we can only say that its apparent harmlessness has not yet been *disproved.*

The problem of the drug's effects on the mind is a very difficult one to dispose of, as so very little is known about its actual operation. The old claim was that cannabis made people "feeble-minded" and "insane". Once again it is apparently true that the heavy hashish user in the East does suffer some long-term psychological damage, but similar evidence in North America is difficult to come by, and much of what there is seems to be circumstantial. Since cannabis users have tended to come from depressed social groups and slum areas, which already possess a relatively high degree of psychological disturbance, it is all too easy for law-enforcement officials to blame the troublesome and rebellious behavior of such persons on the drug rather than on the poverty and repression upon which discontent and disorder grows.

It has been suggested that cannabis use can precipitate a psychosis. Naive users sometimes panic, but experienced users learn how to suppress these effects. Since becoming a pot smoker is almost always a learning process carried out within a group, this danger would seem to be minimized. Allentuck and Bowman maintain that "a characteristic marihuana psychosis does not exist. Marihuana will not produce a psychosis *de novo* in a well-integrated, stable person," but on the other hand, "marihuana may precipitate a psychosis in an unstable, disorganized personality, when it is taken in amounts greater than he can tolerate."[67] There are reports of adverse reactions to cannabis. For example, a recent survey of adverse reactions to LSD in Los Angeles noted a large number of reports on cannabis reactions (1,887 reports from medical doctors and psychiatric personnel over an eighteen-month period).[68] Given the multiple drug use apparently characteristic of most of these persons it might be unwise to put too much trust in such figures. After a thorough survey of all the literature on cannabis and psychosis, Murphy comes to an interesting conclusion.

. . . we have the paradox that although it is well established that cannabis use attracts the mentally unstable . . . the prevalence of *major* mental disorders among cannabis users appears to be little, if any, higher than that in the general population . . . therefore it would appear that true cannabis psychosis must either be very rare indeed, or that it must be substituting for other forms of psychosis. Also, the data raise the question whether the use of cannabis may not be protecting some individuals from a psychosis.[69]

5. *Widespread cannabis use would destroy the moral fabric of our society.* When we come to this argument we may have come to the very quintessence of the opposition to cannabis use. Many of the statements made against cannabis, as against all outlawed drugs, really boil down to the single statement that the use of the drug is *immoral*. It is much more difficult to come to grips with just what constitutes this immorality, since many critics really have no idea beyond the simple conviction that it is supposed to be immoral. But one point upon which very many critics appear to be in increasing agreement is that cannabis use will make people slothful and lethargic and undermine the ethic of hard work upon which our North

American way of life has been built. One American journalist (who by his own account gets stoned on pot frequently) has said that if Horatio Alger had been born next to a field of hemp he never would have made it from office boy to president; instead he would have gone on unemployment relief and just stood around smiling. But the same author, who spent some time riding with the Hell's Angels motorcycle gang, admits that to the Angels, marijuana has been used so often and for so long that they no longer confuse the "mystique" with the real effects. Pot "relaxes" them, but does nothing else.[70] Certainly the Angels could not be accused of being passive and lethargic, although one could accuse them of much else. Similarly, on college campuses there is a certain coincidence between pot smokers and student rebels. A couple of years ago there was apprehension on the part of radicals that pot users were lost to the revolutionary cause, by turning their frustrations inward instead of expressing them politically. Some do use cannabis in this way, but with many others, its steady use does not seem to have induced passivity at all. In the East, heavy hashish use is often associated with sloth, but the traditional cultures of these countries are more passive in outlook than ours to begin with, and, moreover, hashish use is concentrated in the lower classes, whose economic outlook is often utterly bleak no matter how much hard work is undertaken.

While there are apparently established cases of permanent drug-induced psychoses, it is perhaps more likely that persons tend to use drugs whose effects tend to agree with the basic personality structure. The Moroccans have a saying that one is a *kif* addict long before one takes one's first pipe. Even if the drug is taken to compensate for certain psychological tendencies, some sort of equilibrium will presumably be sought after. Horatio Alger probably would not have smoked pot even if it grew next door, and if he did it probably would not have done any more than to slightly moderate his fanatical drive for success; it might even have helped him maintain a more balanced personality. The human personality is too complex a structure to be easily turned upside down by the intrusion of a chemical now and again, especially by one whose effects appear to be relatively mild. Secondly, critics who get upset by apparent challenges to the Protestant work ethic are going to have to become accustomed to the fact that with automation and the shift away from a producing to a consuming society, the work ethic is in severe difficulties irrespective of changing fashions in intoxicants. Pot smoking is nothing more than a mere bubble on the surface of a vast transformation of society away from human labor toward machine labor. Obviously the young are adapting more quickly since they have fewer preconceptions about human behavior. To place the 'blame' for these changing values on cannabis is about as sensible a response as to place the blame for the Industrial Revolution on the introduction of tobacco into the Western world. It must also be recognized that to a limited extent, cannabis may be a more appropriate type of intoxicant for a post-industrial society of leisure than alcohol. At the very least it should be admitted that the introduction of any new drug is far more likely to be a symptom rather than a cause of changing values.

In summary we can say that the arguments put forward by opponents of cannabis use are often overdrawn and sometimes baseless. On the other hand it is not possible to completely disregard some of the points made. Unfortunately, legitimate warnings have too often been buried within an overall approach characterized by ignorance, hysteria, self-righteousness, and a brutal authoritarianism toward any who would disagree. The great marijuana scare is a case study in how *not* to wage a campaign against drug use. Most unfortunately of all, many young persons (as well as some not so young) have made the wholly illogical deduction that the exposure of lies and distortions on the part of the opponents of cannabis constitutes in itself an argument *in favor* of using the drug. The sheer idiocy of such a conclusion cannot be overemphasized. There has been a good deal of rubbish propagated about the horrors of heroin: to reject this misinformation does not mean that one ought to rush out and take a shot of heroin.

There are some who deeply believe that cannabis is not only harmless but of great benefit to humanity. Some of these claims are advanced rationally and with moderation. Some advocates possess a kind of crazed messianic mission to convert the heathen, to turn everybody *on*. These latter we might refer to as the Crackpots. They are more or less the exact equivalent of the anti-weed crusaders and the cops, who possess an equally crazed desire to turn everybody *off*, at all costs. The ordinary non-aligned person in the middle must begin to feel like a tap, being alternately switched on and off by two struggling lunatics. We should, however, take the time to deal with some of the pro-cannabis arguments.

1. *Cannabis enhances creativity.* This is an old and familiar

argument, dating from the time when marijuana was associated with Negro jazz music, and taking on new dimensions with contemporary pop culture. There is not the slightest doubt that many, if not most, rock groups smoke pot and some musicians go so far as to maintain that pot helps them both to create and to perform their music. While there is no scientific proof for such a claim – in fact the evidence is that by objective standards performance declines – artistic creativity is a notoriously difficult quality to test. To the extent that cannabis alters the individual's state of consciousness, it may help open perspectives previously closed, and the disorganizing effect of cannabis upon the thought processes may allow certain innovative relationships to be glimpsed. Creative artists have always been fascinated by different states of consciousness; present interest in cannabis is thus neither new nor alarming. The greatest danger is the confusion of the meaningful impact of the drug's effects on the creative mind on the one hand, and the fallacious notion that the creativity is inherent in the *drug* rather than the person. The medieval alchemists knew better than this: to get gold, they said, you must already have gold. It would be foolish either to deny or to exaggerate the creative potential of cannabis. Many other drugs have been used for exactly the same purposes, and probably with as good results. Omar Khayyam lived in an Islamic country but derived his poetic inspiration not from hashish but from wine. *Chacun à son goût.*

A sane society would let its artists alone, to inspire or waste themselves as they see fit. Dylan Thomas drank himself to death, but without alcohol he might never have written the poetry he did. The Chinese poet Li Po crossed a lake late at night after drinking much wine. Seeing the reflection of the moon in the water, he was so moved by its beauty that he leaned out of the boat to kiss the silvery image – and drowned. No one but a drunken poet would do such a thing, but only a drunken poet could have written as well as he did. And besides, it was an exquisite end.

The only really objectionable point about the use of drugs to enhance creativity, is when the audience is informed that a work of art can only be appreciated if the audience is taking the same drug. This is not only an intolerable conceit on the part of the artist but is really a suggestion that the work is not of lasting value on its own merits. There is a new form of intellectual snobbery afoot today that says that unless you turn on with pot you just cannot judge the offerings of contemporary pop culture. When the Beatles' movie

Yellow Submarine began showing in North America there were thinly veiled suggestions in some reviews that if you were not one of the elite who had smoked pot, there was just no way you could really understand the film. This is to degrade art to the level of a course in pharmacology.

2. *Cannabis makes everybody loving.* There really seems to be very little evidence to support such a generalization. It is doubtful that cannabis causes peaceful people to become suddenly violent; it is no less doubtful that it causes violent people to become suddenly peaceful. The elaborate social rituals that have been built up around pot parties are of a kind that encourage friendly interaction: passing a single cigarette around from person to person recalls very old patterns of peaceful tribal gatherings. Considering the importance of the setting in which cannabis is taken, it is easy to see how the circumstances of its use have been mistaken for its intrinsic effects. In such contexts it *may* encourage feelings of love and tranquillity. But it certainly does not have that effect universally. Take the motorcycle gangs, for instance.

3. *Cannabis reveals the infinite.* Hashish has some of the same effects as LSD. In a later chapter we will take a close look at the relationship between drugs and mystical experiences. But the usual run of North American marijuana is so mild and filled with so many impurities that one would have to be a pretty freaky individual to start with, if one were to regularly get mystical experiences on pot.

Like any other intoxicant, cannabis no doubt has its social uses. But when an intoxicant is legal, like alcohol, nobody wastes much time writing books in its praise. We very much need a calm perspective on the whole matter: the opponents and the champions of the drug are at least in full agreement that their subject is of great importance, but it is precisely on this point that the rest of us might beg to disagree. As Yale psychologist and observer of youth, Kenneth Keniston has said: "There isn't any evidence that people are any smarter or more beautiful or wiser taking pot, but there's a lot of evidence that they feel that way."[71] Murphy closes his survey of the scientific literature on cannabis with a very interesting and useful analogy to alcohol.

> Both in the complexity of its effects and in more specific characteristics, cannabis is much closer to alcohol than to the opiates or to cocaine. Like alcohol, it appears to have no deleterious effect on the moderate

user, who knows the correct amount for obtaining relaxation or euphoria without additional effects. As with alcohol, single doses given to naive, unstable subjects can produce an acute confusion, perhaps with violence, while the long-term use of heavy doses can probably lead to partial dementia or to an organic reaction type psychosis. Like alcohol, it is alleged to carry no danger for the stable personality, but to attract the neurotic and psychopathic, who are also the people that tend to take the heavy doses. Neither drug has a significant tendency to produce physical dependence; neither drug leads to withdrawal symptoms under normal conditions; and in neither case does desired dosage tend to increase with time. Finally, where the drugs are not prohibited, society's attitude towards the deteriorated chronic user is in both instances one of great tolerance.[72]

Is cannabis a dangerous drug? The controversy always seems to come down to this question, and the answer is not difficult to find. Of course it is a dangerous drug. *But it cannot be emphasised too often that any drug that affects the central nervous system is dangerous.* Any drug that alters consciousness can become an unhealthy alternative to reality, or can make for unpredictable and possibly dangerous behavior. By the same token, any drug that fails to do these things will not be widely used. There is simply no easy way out of this dilemma. If we assume that cannabis must be banned if it is 'dangerous' then we must also consider the prohibition of alcohol. The question ought to be rephrased to read *"how dangerous is cannabis?"* and when put in this way we might suggest that the mild North American variety could probably be accommodated within a society that tolerates alcohol. Compared to a lot of other possible intoxicants, North American marijuana would appear to be one of the milder and more manageable. This statement does not apply to hashish, however, which may be far more dangerous.

The psychological and physical dangers of using cannabis in our society are only part of the dangers and, indeed, the lesser part. Far more dangerous to the individual than the drug is the law and its enforcement. It is to this, the most unpleasant aspect of cannabis use, to which we must now turn.

Footnotes

[1]Harry J. Anslinger and Fulton Ourslers, *The Murderers* (New York, Farrar, Strauss & Cudahy, 1961), p. 38.

[2]E. R. Bloomquist, *Marijuana* (Beverly Hills, Calif., Glencoe Press, 1968), pp. 1-16.

[3]Norman Taylor, *Narcotics: Nature's Dangerous Gifts* (New York, Dell, 1966), pp. 20-21.

[4]W. Reininger, "Historical Notes," in David Solomon, ed., *The Marihuana Papers* (New York, Signet Books, 1968), pp. 141-42.

[5]*The Travels of Marco Polo*, trans. by Ronald Latham (Harmondsworth, Middlesex, Penguin Books, 1958), pp. 40-42.

[6]Bernard Lewis, "The Assassins: an Historical Essay," *Encounter*, vol. XXIX, no. 5 (November, 1967), p. 39.

[7]Charles Baudelaire, *Les Paradis Artificiels*, précédé de *La pipe d'opium, le hachich, le club des hachichins* par Théophile Gauthier (Paris, Firmin-Didot, 1961), pp. 37-38. (my own translation)

[8]*Ibid.*, pp. 122-23.

[9]*Ibid.*, p. 127.

[10]Selections from all these writers can be found in David Ebin, ed., *The Drug Experience* (New York, Orion Press, 1961), pp. 41-84.

[11]Harry J. Anslinger and C. R. Cooper, "Marijuana: Assassin of Youth," *American Magazine*, vol. CXXIV, no. 19 (July, 1937).

[12]Howard S. Becker, "The Marihuana Tax Act" in Becker, *Outsiders: Studies in the Sociology of Deviance* (New York, Glencoe, 1963). Reprinted in Solomon, *op. cit.*, pp. 94-102. See also Donald T. Dickson, "Bureaucracy and Morality: an Organizational Perspective on a Moral Crusade," *Social Problems*, vol. XVI, no. 2 (Fall, 1968), and Joseph Oteri and Harvey Silverglate, "In the Marketplace of Free Ideas: a Look at the Passage of the Marihuana Tax Act," in J. L. Simmons, ed., *Marihuana: Myths and Realities* (North Hollywood, Calif., Brandon House, 1967), pp. 136-62.

[13]William S. Burroughs, *Naked Lunch* (New York, Grove Press, 1966), p. 134.

[14]Quoted in Alfred R. Lindesmith, *The Addict and the Law* (New York, Vintage Books, 1967), p. 231.

[15]Robert S. de Ropp, *The Master Game: Pathways to Higher Consciousness Beyond the Drug Experience* (New York, Delta, 1968), pp. 36 and 40.

[16]13-14 George V (1923), c. 22, Schedule.

[17]Emily Murphy, *The Black Candle* (Toronto, Thomas Allen, 1922), pp. 331-37.

[18]22-23 George V (1932), c. 20, s. 3 (a).

[19]10 George VI (1946), c. 11, s. 4.

[20]House of Commons, *Debates* (1938), p. 2772.

[21]19-20 George V, c. 49, s. 4.

[22]House of Commons, *Debates* (1938), p. 772.

[23]*Ibid.*, p. 773.

[24]Report of the Indian Hemp Drug Commission (Simla, India, 1894), quoted in Taylor, *op. cit.*, p. 26.

[25]Taylor, *loc. cit.*

[26]*Ibid.*, p. 30.

[27]*New York Daily Worker* (Dec. 28, 1940), quoted in The Mayor's Committee on Marihuana, *The Marihuana Problem in the City of New York: Sociological, Medical, Psychological and Pharmacological Studies* (Lancaster, Pennsylvania, Jacques Cattell Press, 1944), pp. 4-5. This report is most readily available in Solomon, *Marihuana Papers, op. cit.*, and for this reason further references to the report will be to Solomon.

[28]Robert P. Walton, *Marihuana: America's New Drug Problem* (Philadelphia, Lippincott, 1938).

[29]J. F. Siler *et al.*, "Marihuana Smoking in Panama," *The Military Surgeon,* vol. 73 (1933), p. 278.

[30]James M. Phalen, "The Marijuana Bugaboo," *The Military Surgeon,* vol. 93 (1943), pp. 94-95.

[31]E. Marcovitz and H. J. Meyers, "The Marihuana Addict in the Army," *War Medicine,* vol. 6 (1944), pp. 382-91, and S. Charen, and L. Perelman, "Personality Studies of Marihuana Addicts," *American Journal of Psychiatry,* vol. 102 (1946), pp. 674-82. Both studies cited in H. B. M. Murphy, "The Cannabis Habit: a Review of Psychiatric Literature," *Addictions,* vol. 13, no. 1 (Spring, 1966), pp. 3-21.

[32]Mayor's Committee, in Solomon, *op. cit.,* p. 307.

[33]*Ibid.,* p. 331.

[34]*Ibid.,* p. 332.

[35]*Ibid.,* p. 338.

[36]*Ibid.,* p. 363.

[37]*Ibid.,* p. 388.

[38]*Ibid.,* p. 394.

[39]*Ibid.,* p. 408.

[40]F. Ames, "A Clinical and Metabolic Study of Acute Intoxication with Cannabis Sativa and its Role in the Model Psychoses," *Journal of Mental Science,* vol. 104 (October, 1958), pp. 972-99. R. J. Bouquet, "Cannabis," *Bulletin on Narcotics,* vol. 3, no. 1 (1951), pp. 22-43. William McGlothlin, "Toward a Rational View of Marihuana" in J. L. Simmons, ed., *op. cit.,* pp 163-214.

[41]Murphy, *op. cit.,* p. 4.

[42]*Ibid.,* p. 5.

[43]A. T. Weil, N. E. Zinberg, J. M. Nelsen, "Clinical and Psychological Effects of Marihuana in Man," *Science,* vol. 162, no. 3859 (Dec. 13, 1968), pp. 1234-42. The experiment is also described more briefly by Zinberg and Weil in "Cannabis: the First Controlled Experiment," *New Society,* no. 329 (Jan. 16, 1969).

[44]C. L. Scheckel *et al.,* "Behavioral Effects in Monkeys of Racemates of two Biologically Active Marijuana Constituents," *Science,* vol. 160 (June 28, 1968), pp. 1467-69.

[45]Howard S. Becker, "Becoming a Marihuana User," *American Journal of Sociology,* vol. LIX (November, 1953), pp. 235-42. Reprinted in Becker, *Outsiders, op. cit.*

[46]I. C. Chopra and R. N. Chopra, "The use of Cannabis Drugs in India," *Bulletin on Narcotics,* no. 1 (1957), pp. 4-29.

[47]S. Allentuck and K. M. Bowman, "The Psychiatric Aspects of Marihuana Intoxication," *American Journal of Psychiatry,* vol. 99, no. 2 (Sept., 1942), pp. 248-51. Reprinted in Solomon, *op. cit.,* pp. 411-16.

[48]H. L. Freedman and M. J. Rockmore, "Marihuana, Factor in Personality Evaluation and Army Maladjustment," *Journal of Clinical Psychopathology,* vol. 7 (1946), pp. 765-82, vol. 8, pp. 231-36.

[49]United States Government, Presidential Commission on Law Enforcement and the Administration of Justice, *Task Force Report: Narcotics and Drug Abuse* (Washington, D.C., U.S. Government Printing Office, 1967).

[50]H. B. M. Murphy, *op. cit.*, p. 10.

[51]McGlothlin, *op. cit.*, p. 175.

[52]Nicholas Wade, "Pot and Heroin," *New Society*, no. 330 (Jan. 23, 1969), pp. 117-18.

[53]John C. Ball *et al.*, "The Association of Marihuana Smoking with Opiate Addiction in the United States," *Journal of Criminal Law, Criminology, and Police Science*, vol. 59, no. 2 (June, 1968), pp. 171-82.

[54]Lauretta Bender, cited in Murphy, *op. cit.*, p. 24.

[55]H. Blumer *et al.*, "The World of Youthful Drug Use," ADD Center Project, Final Report (Berkeley, University of California Press, 1967).

[56]Earle Albert Rowell and Robert Rowell, *On the Trail of Marihuana, the Weed of Madness* (1939), quoted in Lindesmith, *op. cit.*, p. 232.

[57]*Loc. cit.*

[58]"Girl gets four years for selling heroin," *Globe and Mail* (March 5, 1969).

[59]W. Bromberg, "Marihuana Intoxication," *American Journal of Psychiatry*, vol. 91 (1934), pp. 303-30. And "Marihuana: a Psychiatric Study," *Journal of the American Medical Association*, vol. 113 (1939), pp. 4-12.

[60]O. Moraes Andrade, "The Criminogenic Action of Cannabis (Marihuana) and Narcotics," *Bulletin on Narcotics*, vol. 16, no. 4 (1964), pp. 23-28.

[61]McGlothlin, *op. cit.*, pp. 192-93.

[62]H. B. M. Murphy, *op. cit.*, p. 6.

[63]Blumer *et al.*, *op. cit.*

[64]President's Commission on Law Enforcement, *op. cit.*

[65]R. N. Chopra & G. S. Chopra, "The Present Position of Hemp-Drug Addiction in India" (1939), cited in McGlothlin, *op. cit.*, pp. 176-77, and in H. B. M. Murphy, *op. cit.*, p. 11.

[66]Freedman and Rockmore, *op. cit.*

[67]Allentuck and Bowman, *op. cit.*, pp. 413-14.

[68]J. T. Ungerleider *et al.*, "A Statistical Survey of Adverse Reactions to LSD in Los Angeles County," *American Journal of Psychiatry*, vol. 25, no. 3 (Sept. 1968), pp. 352-57.

[69]H. B. M. Murphy, *op. cit.*, p. 14.

[70]Hunter S. Thompson, *Hell's Angels: the Strange and Terrible Saga of the Outlaw Motorcycle Gangs* (New York, Ballantine Books, 1967), pp. 271-72.

[71]*Newsweek* (July 24, 1967), p. 50.

[72]H. B. M. Murphy, *op. cit.*, p. 19.

Chasing the Weed

5

There are two subcultures among prisoners today: the criminal and delinquent, and the marijuana users.

Assistant Director of Corrections for
British Columbia (May, 1969).

John Lennon once described cannabis as a "harmless giggle," but when he was arrested and convicted of possession it turned out to be neither harmless nor a giggle. Lennon happens to be one of the more prominent victims of the laws against cannabis, but there are thousands less well known all over Canada, the United States and Britain who have found out just what the state will do to 'protect' people from themselves.

André Grandbois was twenty-four years old, with a grade-five education, and homeless in Montreal. During the spring and summer of 1968 two undercover RCMP agents, posing as hippies, met Grandbois. Grandbois sold a cube of hashish to one of these agents for seven dollars at the latter's request. He was arrested and sentenced to two years in St. Vincent de Paul penitentiary. In sentencing Grandbois the judge made it very clear just what real issues were at stake.

The hippies never cease to affirm that they do not disturb anyone, that they lead a peaceful existence, that each individual has the right to live his life as he wishes. The Court does not share in this opinion . . . because any life within a society requires an active and constructive participation on the part of the individuals the society is composed of.

At a time when, in Canada and more than ever in Quebec, everyone is convinced that more and more advanced education is required for facing life and when enormous amounts of money are invested on this basis, these young hippies decide to do nothing, permit themselves to criticize everything, live in unhealthy environments, look for euphoria through the absorption of narcotics, traffic in narcotics and affirm that consuming marihuana or hashish is not unhealthy *per se* and that they are free to dispose of their life and their persons as they see fit.

The Court can only condemn the deplorable way of life which these young people have adopted and it is convinced that there is a direct relationship between the absorption of these narcotics and this way of life. . . .[1]

For the crime of coming from a background of poverty and opting out of what many responsible people call the 'rat race', André Grandbois will spend two years in prison, surrounded by hardened criminals. Anybody who knows anything about our Canadian prisons could hardly imagine a worse environment in which to place anyone who is supposed to be 'rehabilitated'. And yet the Canadian courts have gone into the business of sending large numbers of young people like Grandbois to spend lengthy periods in such institutions.

A young student at a Canadian university spent a summer in Israel and brought back some hashish with him, for which he was later arrested. A few days before his trial, the Minister of National Health and Welfare made a speech in which he expressed some concern over the imposition of criminal records on young people who would never otherwise have such records, and suggested that the Government was willing to reconsider the legal status of marijuana offences. The judge who considered the case went out of his way to criticize those who minimized the seriousness of narcotics offences, and then sentenced the defendant to a year and a half in prison. How many people can seriously believe that to wreck a young man's university studies and to hang a prison record around his neck for the rest of his life will in any way 'help' him?

K. is twenty-five years old. Two years ago he was asked by a friend to pick up some pot. Five dollars was exchanged, the 'friend' turned out to be an undercover cop, and K. was sentenced to six months in prison. Upon release he decided that he could not take another such ordeal and so gave up both pot and his friends. After trying for some months he got a job. When his 'record' for 'dope-peddling' was revealed, he was fired. He is wondering now how many times this will be repeated in the future. Perhaps he is already wondering what is the use. Score another victory for law and order.

Cases like those above could be multiplied *ad nauseam*. It is possible to state quite unequivocally that any personal dangers associated with marijuana use are quite miniscule compared to the dangers associated with the law. Recalling that objective, scientific tests have indicated that marijuana is a mild intoxicant, which usually brings about a slight euphoria, a slowing of the time sense, a sharpening of the appetite, and perhaps a pleasingly languid appreciation of the senses, it is altogether astonishing to realize what the law prescribes for such forbidden pleasures.

The law makes no distinction of any kind between heroin, morphine, and opium on the one hand, and cannabis on the other. Nor does it make any distinction between the hashish and the marijuana forms of cannabis. In an earlier chapter we have already discussed at some length the provisions of the *Narcotic Control Act* of 1961, but we can recapitulate some of the more alarming features. For possessing marijuana one is subject to seven years in prison; for trafficking one can be imprisoned for life. For importing the drug one cannot be sentenced to less than seven years; life imprisonment is the maximum. Cultivating the cannabis plant carries a maximum sentence of seven years. A second offence for trafficking or importing can bring about a sentence of preventive detention for an indeterminate period. Under the Act, police officers can be issued with special Writs of Assistance that allow them to enter any dwelling house at any time to search for narcotics. In the course of such searches, officers may break open any object in the house. If charged with possession, the accused is considered guilty until he can prove to the Court that he is innocent. If charged with possession for the purpose of trafficking, he must first prove that he was not in possession. If he fails to prove this to the Court's satisfaction, he is then considered guilty of possession for the purpose of trafficking unless he is able to prove otherwise.

And all this for the 'crime' of smoking a weed that has been used by countless millions of human beings for five thousand years or more! It is truly astonishing. Especially in a country that prides itself on its alleged sense of justice and fair play, and that proudly tells its children that the police can only enter a private home with a search warrant, and that a defendant is always assumed to be innocent until proven guilty. It is no less astonishing that the same Government that passed the *Narcotic Control Act* also passed the *Canadian Bill of Rights*.

On one important point, Canadian legislation is much superior to

American legislation. Except for importing, there are no mandatory minimum sentences prescribed. It is on this basis that judicial flexibility in sentencing is possible and a consequent *de facto* distinction between the seriousness of opiate and marijuana offences, which the law itself does not recognize. Statistical analysis of all sentences for possession offences concerning marijuana and all sentences involving possession of heroin done by the Addiction Research Foundation of Ontario has shown a steady trend toward suspended sentences and probation for marijuana offenders compared to a continuous pattern of prison sentences for heroin violators.[2] Unfortunately such a trend is only a general statistical movement. Some judges do not believe in leniency and so to the 'lottery' aspect of arrests for marijuana, one must add a lottery aspect to sentencing. In one Canadian city, for example, it is an open secret that if a marijuana offender comes before one particular judge he has a chance for some sympathy; if he is unfortunate enough to come before a certain other judge, however, the penitentiary is almost a certainty. Some judges are genuinely confused and seek advice. Others are apparently quite single-minded in applying the letter of the law. Faced with the unsettling phenomenon of large numbers of young people – many of whom are from 'respectable' middle-class homes – suddenly appearing before the courts, neither the courts themselves nor the Federal Justice Department have been able to establish a clear and consistent sentencing strategy.

In 1967 an eighteen year old first offender convicted on five counts of trafficking in marijuana in the Yorkville district of Toronto, was given a two year suspended sentence by a local magistrate on condition that he keep away from Yorkville friends, live at home with his parents, obey a ten p.m. curfew, return to school, and take psychiatric treatment. The Federal Justice Department appealed this sentence as being too lenient. The Ontario Court of Appeal upheld the magistrate's decision, on the grounds that the defendant represented a new social phenomenon in Canada, a trafficker in drugs who is neither an addict nor a profit-seeker, but who instead views the use of drugs as socially desirable. The Court felt that a "deterrent" type of sentence would only confirm such persons in their beliefs, and quite frankly admitted that this was a new social problem the solution of which was not yet known.[3]

While this decision seemed to have signalled a more realistic approach, it was not a direction generally followed. In the same year a twenty-three year old M.A. student in psychology and teaching assistant at the University of Alberta was convicted of possession of marijuana. A sentence of one day was appealed by the Federal government and in the Alberta Supreme Court was changed to a sentence of three months. The Government argued that the original sentence had failed to take into account the "ascendancy in the hierarchy of crime" of offences involving narcotics, as well as the need for deterrence and rehabilitation. In its judgment, the Court also brought another factor into consideration, that of retribution.[4]

In January of 1968 the same Ontario court that had five months earlier upheld the suspended sentence referred to previously, seemed to have changed its mind by sentencing an eighteen year old trafficker to nine months definite and six months indefinite. They noted that the traffic in marijuana had markedly increased since the previous case had been decided, and they now stressed the value of deterrent sentences, and specifically stated that the social views of marijuana users did not entitle them to any special treatment.[5]

Almost simultaneous with this judgment was the case of R. v. Adelman in British Columbia. Morley Adelman was a twenty-five year old graduate student with an outstanding academic record. He was given a suspended sentence for possession of marijuana. This sentence was appealed by the Justice Department in the British Columbia Court of Appeal and changed to six months. In its judgment, the Court made it clear that students and intellectuals

. . . by reason of their intelligence should know better. They should appreciate by reason of their training that the laws of the country have to be respected and upheld and obeyed, even though the individual person may not agree with them.
. . . A person of superior education and intelligence is, to my mind, *more blameworthy* than the less fortunate individual with little education or dull intellect. The former ought to know better than to deliberately disobey the law and so set a bad example to others. He deserves *a more severe penalty* than the latter.[6] (emphasis added)

At about the time of the Adelman decision it became generally known that the Federal government intended to demand jail terms for young first offenders. The Toronto *Globe and Mail* suggested that this get-tough policy was

. . . an accurate reflection of the abiding faith that Canada has traditionally had in prison sentences. At the most recent count our jail population had declined slightly, but it was still large enough to proclaim the general inclination of our system of law to prescribe prison as the all-purpose medicine to cure our social ills.

This is the blindest kind of faith, and it is a particularly foolish philosophy to apply to first offenders in cases of possessing marijuana. One need not approve the use of marijuana by young people to recognize the difference between an experimenter and a criminal.[7]

This was not the view of the Government. On March 21, 1968, Mr. Pierre Elliott Trudeau (then the Minister of Justice) told the House of Commons that his department, if asked for guidance by the courts in sentencing, would suggest that the Adelman case be used as a model and that sentences and fines ordinarily be imposed as deterrents.[8]

In Manitoba later that year, a twenty year old student named McNichol was convicted and sentenced to one month in jail. The Crown appealed and the Court of Appeal imposed a one year sentence. The magistrate in the original decision had been concerned lest the defendant's studies should suffer. The Court of Appeal had no such scruples, however, and castigated the magistrate for being "much too concerned with the possible rehabilitation of this young offender. . . . In doing so he completely disregarded the interests of the community and put those of the individual ahead of the community."[9] This constitutes one of the clearest statements on record of the doctrine of majoritarian conservatism in a judicial guise.

Although it is still too early to tell, the trend in 1969 may be away from punitive sentences. In November of 1968, the British Columbia Court of Appeals apparently modified its own precedent of R. v. Adelman by dismissing an appeal by the Government against a one day and $500 sentence for possession. The Court agreed that "deterrence" was the primary factor to be considered but felt that a prison sentence was not always mandatory, regardless of circumstances.[10] And in December the Manitoba Court of Appeal dismissed a Government appeal that was based upon the same court's McNichol decision. The Court took the opportunity to specifically deny that the McNichol decision had bound the Court to use prison sentences as the only answer.

As a summary of these cases indicates, the judicial policy in sentencing has been anything but clear and consistent. With the general recognition on the part of the Federal government that deterrence is not working there may be a change toward more liberal sentencing patterns. The only general conclusion that can be drawn is that when thousands of young people begin appearing in the courts charged under an Act that assumes that the offence is so serious that it must be treated in a manner that would be considered contrary to our basic freedoms even in a case of murder, and when at the same time the 'criminals' in question are the sort who would never otherwise be in court, and when, to make matters even more complicated, there is a raging debate in the society at large as to whether the behavior in question ought to be considered criminal at all – when all these factors come together at once, then the machinery of justice starts to come apart. There are undoubtedly a number of very perplexed and bewildered judges in Canada today who simply lack any guidelines to deal with such cases. As one magistrate frankly admitted, "the Courts desperately need scientific guidance in assessing the marijuana problem."[11]

Thankfully, neither our Canadian legislators nor our judges have shown the extreme bloodthirstiness displayed by some American legislators and judges. In Colorado a second offence for the sale of marijuana to anyone under twenty-five could be punished by death in the gas chamber; although such a penalty has never been invoked, it stands as a grisly monument to a law run amok. But the sentences handed down are chilling enough. On the night of his twenty-second birthday, Kerrigan Gray, a student in the State of Washington was arrested for having sold an amount of marijuana to an undercover narcotics agent posing as a student. This agent had become friends with Gray and asked him to procure some pot. Gray obliged his 'friend' and for this act was sentenced to twenty years in the state prison, the first fourteen months of which were spent in maximum security. Timothy Leary, the so-called high priest of LSD, was arrested when crossing the border from Mexico to Texas and convicted of being in possession of less than one-half ounce of marijuana. For this Leary was sentenced to thirty years imprisonment, along with a $30,000 fine. On May 19, 1969, this conviction was overturned by the United States Supreme Court, which ruled that certain provisions of the *Marihuana Tax Act* are unconstitutional. The principle of laws prohibiting the use of cannabis was not, however, called into question by this decision and it is to be expected that new federal legislation will be drafted to accomplish the same purpose as the old.

Even if Canadian laws are less rigid in sentencing procedures –

under American federal law a first offence for selling marijuana carries with it a mandatory minimum sentence of five years, and possession two years – nevertheless Canadian law is just as firmly founded on the same assumptions as the United States laws: namely that marijuana represents a grave and imminent threat to the well-being of our society, and that the best way to combat this menace is to employ stiff prison sentences as deterrents.

That is the theory behind the law. We have already suggested that the first premise is grotesque when placed against the sound scientific evidence of the effects of marijuana. The second premise has already been proven false. In 1963 marijuana offences constituted a tiny proportion of all offences under the *Narcotic Control Act*. In 1967 there were 586 convictions for marijuana offences. In 1968 this figure had jumped to 1,429. Nine out of ten persons convicted on marijuana charges in 1968 were under 25 years of age, and three out of five were under 21.[12] Marijuana violations now far exceed heroin offences and the trend is upward. The theory of deterrence has proven to be about as effective as the American policy of bombing North Vietnam.

When the law tries to ban the sale and use of some commodity or service, but people continue to buy and use the commodity, the net effect is usually a form of government *regulation* of the market. Since punitive laws, deterrent sentences, and zealous police enforcement have failed not only to eradicate the use of marijuana but have even failed to prevent its widespread proliferation, we must examine the *practice* of the law, as well as the theory to determine what effect the law has had in regulating the conditions of sale of marijuana.

The first point is that of quality control. As the drug is illegal there is no way that the buyer can be protected by inspection of the content of the marijuana sold. When we buy a bottle of liquor we know exactly what we are getting because the dosage of ethyl alcohol is clearly labelled on the outside. The pot smoker buys an unknown commodity. He may be paying for oregano or green tea or crushed basil leaves or even catnip. He may be getting a large proportion of material from the inactive male plant. All this will be quite harmless, although a waste of money. But there are reports of toxic impurities being found in marijuana, and reports of bad reactions on the part of smokers who are quite capable of handling marijuana, as such. There are also reports of distributors mixing heroin with marijuana in order to hook young people on hard narcotics.[13] Some regular users express great concern about this. Actually, this fear may be very exaggerated. It is doubtful, medically, that persons can become addicted to heroin unknowingly or unwittingly as we pointed out earlier when discussing the psychology of addiction (Chapter 2).

This also brings up another point. In order to produce and distribute an illegal commodity an illegal sales network is necessary, as well as a subculture of drug users. In such an environment both profit motives and social values encourage multiple drug use. Pot smokers may take LSD, or take amphetamines and become speed freaks. It is my impression that most of the traffic in marijuana is still in the hands of young people. But even here there is a strong incentive to try other, more dangerous, hallucinogenics and amphetamine drugs. The more the laws are enforced, the more the traffic is harassed, the higher the prices become and the more incentive there is for organized criminal elements to move in on the market – and the more likely it is that heroin will be made available. A moralistic law thus turns out in practice to have a quite different effect than that intended by its framers.

A particularly distasteful aspect of the marijuana law situation is the use of police undercover agents to infiltrate groups of young marijuana users and to entrap them into selling some drugs. There is something very unedifying about an agent posing as a youth's friend or associate and instigating a criminal offence for which the unfortunate youth may pay dearly. There are very real questions of public morality involved in this matter, particularly when some testimony has indicated that on occasion the agent has persistently sought to make a purchase from an unwilling source. Should an action undertaken to oblige a friend be placed on the same legal footing as a carefully planned criminal operation undertaken for personal gain? An exceptionally revolting use of undercover agents occurred at Cornell University in New York State, where an agent posing as a student actually conducted an affair with a girl who, upon complying with her boyfriend's request for some pot, was promptly arrested. She was eventually acquitted, but on a legal technicality, not on the gross immorality of the police behavior. Not surprisingly there is a good deal of paranoia afoot among youth about the activities of the "narcs". When even high school students begin seeing police spies behind every telephone pole we have gone a long way down the road to a police state. And what is the net effect of all these activities? After a few months of undercover activity there is a grand bust and a number of bedraggled hippies are thrown into jail. The newspapers are full of headlines that proclaim DOPE RING SMASHED or NARCOTICS RAID NETS HIPPIE DRUG PEDDLERS. Out in the suburbs, Mr. and Mrs. Middle-Class Canada go to bed feeling safer that night. And meanwhile the number of pot smokers continues to increase as if nothing had happened.

A new twist to the scene has been added by attempts to encourage parents to turn their children in to the police if they find drugs in their possession. According to a newspaper report, "In Seattle, the police encourage parents to provide information that would be useful in prosecuting their children and even to testify against them in court. Many parents co-operate 'because they feel what's right is right', a police spokesman said."[14] In Ottawa recently a teen-age girl was turned in by her parents when a small amount of hashish was found in her room. The magistrate commended them for their "concern" for their "daughter's welfare," and their "faith in our legal system". Parents ought to be aware that they are doing their children far more lasting harm by offering them up on the bloody altar of an insane law. Children who become involved in drugs may well need help, but help is the last thing that the law, in its present state, can offer. You do not cure your child's infected finger by chopping off his hand.

Perhaps the most disturbing aspect of the entire situation is the extent to which marijuana laws are, or can be used as, a means of political repression. Many people smoke pot. But if you are an older middle-class or a professional person you have almost nothing to fear from the law. If you are a so-called hippie or if you have done anything to attract attention to yourself in a political sense, the laws against marijuana are a handy instrument that the State can employ as a means of repression. In Buffalo, a leading American literary critic, Leslie Fiedler, was charged with maintaining premises upon which marijuana was smoked. The bust was obviously a set-up and Fiedler never went to jail, but the circumstances surrounding the event were extremely unsettling. Fiedler, who does not smoke pot, had agreed to act as faculty adviser to a student organization promoting the legalization of marijuana. The fraudulent charges were clearly an attempt to intimidate Fiedler as well as the students from employing what is supposed to be a constitutional right to freedom of speech.[15]

In Britain the summer of 1967 witnessed the great Rolling Stones controversy. The Stones, always the most anarchistic and defiant of pop stars, were probably among the least popular Britons to the middle-aged, and among the most popular to the young. Mick Jagger was charged with having four pep pills – which had been legally prescribed in Italy – and sentenced to three months. Keith Richards, lead guitarist of the group, was sentenced to one year for "permitting his premises to be used for the smoking of cannabis resin" (hashish). These sentences, particularly that of Jagger, roused a great furor. A writer in the *Sunday Times* called it a "case of social revenge".[16] The venerable *Times* devoted a lead editorial to Jagger's sentence under the title of "Who breaks a butterfly on a wheel?" and made the point that "if we are going to make any case a symbol of the conflict between the sound traditional values of Britain and the new hedonism, then we must be sure that the sound traditional values include those of tolerance and equity."[17] It was obvious that the drug charges were only the surface manifestation of a general social disapproval of the Rolling Stones and the way of life they represented. Jagger and Richards were being made examples of, not so much for what they *did* as for what they *were*. Eventually the charges were thrown out, but the bad taste lingers on.

We have not had such spectacular cases in Canada but there are examples none the less of marijuana being used as a pretext for what is essentially a form of *political* repression. In the past few years a number of so-called underground newspapers have sprung up in some major Canadian cities and have uniformly felt the brunt of official disapproval. Charges, ranging from peddling without a licence to obscenity and libel, have been brought against them. In Ottawa a number of attempts were made to stop the publication and distribution of a paper known as the *Ottawa Free Press*.[18] A number of persons associated with the paper have been convicted of various cannabis offences, but in one particular instance, the political overtones became ominous. Photographs obtained by the paper showed a pot bust on the city's downtown shopping mall. The editor's home was soon after entered and searched by RCMP narcotics agents. The editor claimed that in fact the police were looking for the photographs, but charges were later laid under the *Narcotic Control Act*. These charges were not proved in court, but soon after he was arrested again for possession of a large quantity of hashish and sentenced to two years in prison. The case roused considerable local interest and had other repercussions. For example, an administrative employee of the City of Ottawa was dismissed from his job when he criticized the actions of the magistrate.

The point is not that innocent people are being sent to prison on false evidence, but rather that certain vulnerable individuals take the brunt of a law that many are able to violate with relative impunity. It is a sick situation when ninety-nine persons can smoke pot and get away with it while the hundredth – who does smoke pot but who happens also to be a hippie, or a political radical, or an editor of an underground paper – can be given a lengthy prison term. And consider for a moment what such a spectacle does to any lingering respect for law and authority held by young people.

All things considered, it is scarcely surprising that the Great Marijuana Scare has turned into the Great Marijuana Controversy. In the 1930s the public was much readier to accept the word of the authorities about the horrors of the hemp weed. For one thing its use was confined to socially 'undesirable' groups. And perhaps people believed what they were told more readily in those days. Today things are very different. The pot smoker may be Mr. and Mrs. Middle-Class's darling son or daughter. Increasingly it may even be Mr. or Mrs. Middle-Class themselves. We are now informed by *MacLean's Magazine* that "Some of the Best People Smoke Pot."[19] The "best people" turn out, of course, to be nice, clean-cut, responsible, business and professional types, like a Toronto lawyer reputed to stroll through Nathan Phillips Square in Toronto on his lunch hour, puffing pot. (Given the strong and distinctive smell of burning marijuana, I find this story to be somewhat doubtful journalism.)

In July of 1967 a full-page advertisement was placed in the *Times* of London under the heading "the law against marijuana is immoral in principle and unworkable in practice."[20] The advertisement was signed by some sixty-four prominent Britons including members of parliament, fellows of the Royal Society, medical doctors, psychiatrists, and such well-known personalities as novelist Graham Greene, critic Kenneth Tynan, Nobel prize winning biologist Sir Francis Crick, the Beatles, and all-purpose student revolutionary Tariq Ali. It was a glittering cast to be assembled for any cause, and particularly for one as laden with bad associations as the legalization of cannabis use. The advertisement summarized some of the main arguments for allowing the use of cannabis, and quoted Spinoza to the effect that:

All laws which can be violated without doing anyone any injury are laughed at. Nay, so far are they from doing anything to control the desires and passions of man that, on the contrary, they direct and incite men's thoughts toward what is forbidden and desire the things they are not allowed to have. And men of leisure are never deficient in the ingenuity needed to enable them to outwit laws framed to regulate things which cannot be entirely forbidden. . . . He who tries to determine everything by law will foment crime rather than lessen it.

Four years earlier, *The Lancet* – the British medical journal – had suggested in an editorial that putting cannabis on the same legal footing as alcohol was "worth considering". They cited the "undoubted attraction of reducing, for once, the number of crimes that a member of our society can commit," the possible revenue that the State could derive from cannabis sales, and the reduction of tension between the generations.[21] It would seem then that 'respectable' opinion in Britain has expressed itself far more clearly in favor by legalizing cannabis in Britain than it has in either the United States or Canada. But opposition has been equally strong. The former Conservative cabinet minister Quinton Hogg has on a number of occasions publicly delivered himself of the opinion that the *Times* ought never to have even printed the pro-cannabis advertisement, and the continued harassment of the Rolling Stones and the Beatles by the drug squads symbolizes a continuing legal harassment of cannabis users in Britain. The exaggerated fear in which cannabis is held by Western societies is reflected in the peculiar situation in Britain where heroin addiction is treated more lightly by the law than cannabis use. And what is more, the situation is quite unlikely to improve. An official Parliamentary Committee recently investigated the whole question of cannabis, dismissed most of the myths associated with the drug's use, and recommended a considerable liberalization of the laws. The Wooton Report, as it was known, was immediately denounced in the House of Commons not only by Mr. Hogg as opposition spokesman but also by the Labour Home Secretary, Mr. James Callaghan. The latter in fact made it clear that far from liberalizing the law, the Labour government intended to stiffen it considerably.

The prospects for reform have been even dimmer in the United States. Some prominent voices have been raised in opposition to the marijuana myths. Dr. James Goddard, head of the United States

Food and Drug Administration put himself into the centre of a vicious political storm when he publicly stated that "whether or not marijuana is a more dangerous drug than alcohol is debatable. I don't happen to think it is."[22] A psychologist who directs the country's largest federally sponsored drug education project recommended recently that laws against the possession of marijuana be removed. "The assumptions on which the laws were based have one by one been proved incorrect," she said. "I would think that our enforcement agencies and our courts have far more important concerns than marijuana."[23] Studies done for the Task Force on Narcotics and Drug Abuse of the President's Crime Commission in 1967 went a long way toward demonstrating how distorted are many, if not most, official views on cannabis. The radical implications of the Task Force studies were watered down somewhat in the Task Force recommendations, and by the time that the Commission's general recommendations were made, the call for liberalization had been transmuted into a call for strengthening the staff of the Narcotics Bureau, and the government eventually responded with *stiffer* laws. Such is often the fate of reform proposals once they are fed into the bureaucratic process.

Another type of attack is being waged in the United States against the marijuana laws, this time in the courts. Joseph Oteri, a Boston lawyer whose practice is now made up almost entirely of marijuana cases, is challenging the constitutionality of anti-marijuana legislation. The first test came late in 1967 when sentences against two college students were appealed to the Massachusetts Superior Court on the grounds that the laws are "arbitrary, irrational and unsuited to the accomplishment of any valid legislative purpose," and contrary to the Ninth Amendment to the United States Constitution, which guarantees defendants' rights, to the due process and equal protection clauses of the Fourteenth Amendment, and to the prohibition against cruel and unusual punishments guaranteed by the Eighth and Fourteenth Amendments. This appeal involved the hearing of numerous expert witnesses and of conflicting evidence on the values and dangers of marijuana. The appeal was ultimately dismissed. While the constitutional and legal aspects of an American case have little bearing on Canadian law, the judgment touched on one general point in terms very revealing of the establishment attitudes toward cannabis and alcohol. Mr. Chief Justice Tauro, while admitting the dangers of excessive alcohol consumption, maintained that

. . . alcohol has uses other than as a means of becoming intoxicated. The vast majority of alcohol users do not consume it with the intention of becoming intoxicated. It has a social value as a relaxant . . . Marihuana, on the other hand . . . is used solely as a means of intoxication . . . The history and cultural acceptance of alcohol and marihuana in this country cannot be ignored. Alcohol has been in widespread use among the general population since colonial times . . . So ingrained is its use in our culture that all prior statutory and constitutional prohibitions of its use have failed . . . [Marijuana] use was never widespread among the general population . . . Nor has its use become so ingrained in our culture as to make strictly prohibiting its use impractical.[24]

The Women's Christian Temperance Union in Ontario recently announced that public fears about marijuana and LSD were merely a smokescreen to hide the real issue, that of alcohol. In a way they may have had a point. In any event, Mr. Oteri is continuing his legal fight against the marijuana laws, however dim his chances of success in a North America run by an establishment that says alcohol is acceptable because we accept it, but that another drug is unacceptable, because of the fact that we do not accept it – while at the same time thousands of people who *do* accept it are thrown into jail, as a means of proving that the drug is unacceptable. The argument that the value of something is proved by its acceptance while its value is disproved by its non-acceptance is as immobile a piece of reactionary illogic as could be imagined: how, after all, did *alcohol* become accepted in the first place?

The controversies that have been shaking Britain and the United States have not been absent in Canada. Many persons, including members of parliament, judges, and medical and professional figures, have called for a high level investigation of the scientific facts concerning cannabis. Even a former Commissioner of the RCMP has suggested such a study. Clifford W. Harvison told an Ottawa newspaper that "we don't really know what the effects of it are. Perhaps it is harmful, perhaps not. But we can't change the law without knowing exactly what its effects are."[25] In the fall of 1967 a committee of the British Columbia Medical Association proposed that cannabis be distributed in Canada in the same way as alcohol. Pointing out that cannabis is being used in Vancouver by 'squares' from every social and economic stratum of society, who moreover remain economically productive even when cannabis users, and further suggesting that the law, by creating a new class of criminal might thereby be producing "more social disruption than could result from unrestricted use of the drug," the committee therefore proposed that a Government marijuana control board might be a more appropriate legal control than present restrictions. However, the committee's report was rejected by the general assembly of the association after a prolonged debate – although the assembly did suggest that some more appropriate form of control might be sought in place of the present system.[26]

One authoritative voice raised against the present legal status of cannabis is that of Dr. J. Robertson Unwin, Director of the Adolescent Service at the Allan Memorial Institute of Montreal and Assistant Professor of Psychiatry at McGill University. Dr. Unwin surveyed the medical evidence on cannabis and came to the conclusion that the North American variety was a relatively mild drug that should be considered quite separately from other drugs of abuse, and suggested that the marijuana controversy may "eventually be reduced to the issue of civil liberties."[27] In an appearance before a joint committee of the Senate and House of Commons, Dr. Unwin expressed the hope that "consideration will be given soon to removing marijuana from the *Narcotic Control Act* and its possession from the category of criminal offence." He said that making possession of the drug a criminal offence is "starkly unjust in view of the known medical facts." In an interview, Dr. Unwin said he doubts that North American marijuana is as dangerous to health and to society as alcohol. He also cautioned that "it still takes a good deal of courage to make any liberal statement about these drugs in public."[28] The latter point is certainly true. Dr. Joel Fort was fired from his position as head of San Francisco's Center for Special Problems, for moderate statements he made about marijuana use. In California a school principal was fired for publicly stating that she had smoked marijuana for years. Happily we have been largely free from this kind of hysteria in Canada. Dr. Unwin's article on the medical aspects of cannabis use has even been distributed by the Department of National Health and Welfare to interested persons who request information on drugs. It is to be fervently hoped that such an open-minded approach will be continued and even expanded.

The Addiction Research Foundations of British Columbia and

Ontario have been other welcome voices of moderation and good sense in the controversy. Such foundations, relatively independent of both law enforcement agencies and of political influences, have an extremely important role to play in carrying out research, helping drug users who need help and in providing authoritative scientific information for the public. While the Foundations have, quite rightly, emphasized the personal dangers of cannabis use, they have not avoided the legal dangers as well. The Ontario Foundation, for example, in an official statement widely circulated throughout the province, has stated flatly that "most of the problems associated with the occasional moderate use of marihuana arise not from its pharmacological actions, but from the fact that possession of the drug is illegal. It is probably undesirable to subject users of marihuana to the severe penalties that are provided in the narcotics control legislation." The Foundation adds that unless the many unanswered questions about cannabis can be satisfactorily answered, it "would also be undesirable to legalize [its] sale and use."[29] Various persons associated with the Ontario Foundation have publicly reiterated the point that present laws are much too severe.[30] An official of the Foundation has stated publicly that "as far as we know it [marijuana] does no harm."[31] However, the Foundation itself is unlikely to support such a strong stand.

In July of 1968 the John Howard Society of Ontario presented the Minister of Justice with a well-documented brief arguing that penalties for cannabis use be reduced, that a separate cannabis control act be established allowing the Crown to proceed either by summary conviction or by indictment, that wider use of suspended sentences for first offenders be considered, and that concerted research be undertaken into the entire question of cannabis and its effects.[32] The Elizabeth Fry Society and the United Church of Canada have also added their voices to the chorus of protest against the present law.

In 1968 the Minister of National Health and Welfare, John Munro, suggested to the annual convention of the Canadian Pharmaceutical Association in Regina that the Federal government might be considering lowering the penalties for marijuana offences. While ruling out the legal distribution of the drug, he suggested that a teen-ager who tries pot at a Saturday night party might be foolish, but is not, after all, a criminal – and that it makes no sense for the Government to become a mass dispenser of criminal records to curious young people. Reaction from the RCMP and from metropolitan police chiefs across Canada was generally hostile, ranging from Toronto Police Chief James Mackey's comment that to be permissive in drug matters is "just damned nonsense" to Winnipeg's Chief George Blow, who agreed that marijuana should be removed from the narcotics category.

In October of 1968 Mr. Munro announced that steps might be taken to place marijuana within a new category of restricted drugs (along with LSD, STP, and other hallucinogenics), which would be created by an amendment to the *Food and Drugs Act* of 1961. Under this legislation, the Crown would have the option of proceeding either by summary conviction or by indictment. If marijuana were to be put into this category, and if summary convictions were handed down, the person convicted would not necessarily receive a criminal record because local police do not normally take fingerprints to be filed with the RCMP in Ottawa. However, local police do retain records and these could be searched by police in other municipalities.[33] Lower penalties would also result from the inclusion of marijuana in this new category. An examination of the new legislation indicates, however, that many of the most objectionable features of the *Narcotic Control Act* would also apply to the new restricted drug category – the special police powers, Writs of Assistance, and the assumption of the defendant's guilt until he proves his own innocence, would all apply to marijuana offences whether under the old Act or under the new category.[34]

In a later interview Mr. Munro expressed great doubts as to whether legislation is really the answer to drug problems and maintained that the root of the problem is to determine the reasons why young people take drugs.[35]

Despite Mr. Munro's genuine concern, there is powerful opposition to liberalization among both government officials and law enforcement authorities. Eventually in the summer of 1969, the *Narcotic Control Act* was amended so as to allow the Crown the option of proceeding upon summary conviction in cases of possession. Upon summary conviction, a first offence now carries a fine of $1,000 or six months imprisonment, or both; for a subsequent offence, the fine is $2,000 or one year's imprisonment.[36] In other words, the intent of Mr. Munro's earlier suggestion toward liberalizing the treatment of marijuana offences is to be carried within the *Narcotic Control Act*.

Despite the Minister's good intentions, it cannot be said that any significant change has been brought about. As things stand presently, marijuana will continue to be classified (erroneously) as a narcotic along with heroin, morphine, and opium. The lower penalties may not mean very much *in practice* as most sentences for possession of marijuana have tended to be much lighter than the maximum possible. Under summary proceedings, criminal records are not really wiped out but are perhaps at best more easily hidden. One Federal official was quoted as saying that with summary convictions it is "much easier to lie successfully about such a record when applying for a job or a visa."[37] All in all, an examination of the 'reform' of the laws against marijuana would indicate that the actual change is less than meets the eye. In fairness to Mr. Munro, however, it must be noted that a new committee is being set up to undertake a two-year study of drug problems. Perhaps the Government hopes to postpone major changes in the law until they are presented with an informed and independent perspective based on scientific research. But the Government must also remember that the impact of the law is a very immediate and pressing problem to a large number of young people, not to speak of their parents.

We have examined the medical evidence; we have seen the gravity of the law compared to the relative insignificance of the offence; we have seen that many moderate and responsible people have supported some meaningful reform of the law. But one question remains: why does the opposition to change run so deep? In many ways, this is the most difficult question of all to answer.

Conservatism and inertia in the face of a confusing situation probably has a lot to do with it. Ambrose Bierce once defined a conservative as a "statesman who is enamoured of existing evils, as distinguished from the liberal, who wishes to replace them with others". The status quo is always given the benefit of the doubt even when that doubt becomes overwhelming, and, like marijuana offenders, reform proposals are presumed to be guilty until proven innocent. But even if we give an existing law the benefit of the doubt, there can no longer be *any doubt* that the treatment of cannabis offences has failed. It has no effect on the traffic: large numbers of people import, grow, distribute, purchase, and consume marijuana and hashish; only an unlucky few get caught in the law enforcement lottery, and these are treated in a manner quite out of proportion to the offence, and may well be unable to secure jobs, hold public office, or obtain travel visas for the rest of their lives. So long as the defenders of the existing law demand that reform proposals be *proven* to be completely without danger, there will assuredly be no reform. It must be emphasized that in the matter of drugs, there cannot be any perfect solutions. Drug use is itself a symbol of the imperfection of human society and the necessity to have some means of escape from the world that we ourselves have made; but the attempt to utterly eradicate this escape mechanism involves the State in a brutal assault upon human nature itself. Any reform will involve dangers; but the maintenance of the existing situation involves enough known dangers that some attempt at innovation and creativity must be made. Lord Clarendon, a royalist in the English civil war, once said that "when it is not necessary to change, it is necessary not to change." This is a fine conservative principle, but conservatives must accept that in this matter it *is* necessary to change.

The opposition to change is to a considerable extent a symbolic struggle against the values of the young, with the added prize that guilt feelings about adult indulgence in alcohol, tobacco, and pills of all kinds can be projected onto others. By attacking marijuana users, the ordinary citizen proves his own normality and reassures himself that society puts the *imprimateur* of acceptability on his own vices. What is more, stiff anti-marijuana provisions provide a handy weapon for repression of young dissidents who have offended on political or social grounds, without involving the country in messy civil liberties cases.

Speaking from the perspective of the older generation, Robert Fulford sums up exactly the real reasons for the reluctance to entertain change in the cannabis situation.

What we have to come to terms with is that this law — and all the legal apparatus around it — exist only to protect our own vision of society. We grew up knowing a society in which marijuana was seen as an evil thing, an object of horror; and that is the society in which, apparently we prefer to live. To recognize that this situation has changed would threaten us; it might force us to change ourselves; and that, we refuse to do. Therefore, we prefer to maintain the law, and the fiction supporting it. Perhaps, when we come to open the conversation with the young that will be necessary to prevent the breakdown of our society, this fact will be a useful place to begin.[38]

Footnotes

[1]R. v. Grandbois (Jan. 15, 1969), Province of Quebec, District of Montreal. Court of the Sessions of the Peace no. 32213/68. Hon. Justice Jacques Coderre, presiding judge. Typescript copy (translation).

[2]Alcoholism and Drug Addiction Research Foundation, *Seventeenth Annual Report* (1967).

[3]R. v. Hudson (1967) 2 O.R. 501.

[4]R. v. Lehrmann (1967) 61 W.W.R. 625.

[5]R. v. Simpson (1968) 2 O.R. 271.

[6]R. v. Adelman (1968) 63 W.W.R. 294.

[7]"Prison is no panacea," *Globe and Mail* (Feb. 12, 1968).

[8]House of Commons, *Debates* (March 21, 1968), p. 7876.

[9]R. v. McNichol (1968) 1 D.L.R. (3d) 328.

[10]R. v. Reynolds (1969) 66 W.W.R. 767.

[11]"Addict prompts court to lash legal 'pot' bid," *Ottawa Citizen* (Sept. 30, 1968).

[12]Almost three quarters of these convictions were in Ontario (581 or 41%) and British Columbia (426 or 30%). Interestingly enough, 89% of those convicted were male. These calculations are based upon figures supplied by the Department of Justice and the Department of National Health and Welfare.

[13]"Pushers add heroin to marijuana to attract new addicts, MP says," *Globe and Mail* (Nov. 1, 1967).

[14]"Police in two U.S. cities offer free drug analysis," *Globe and Mail* (April 21, 1969).

[15]Leslie Fiedler, "On being busted at fifty," *The New York Review of Books* (July 13, 1967), pp. 8-14.

[16]Hugo Young, "The Stones: a case of social revenge," *The Sunday Times* (July 2, 1967).

[17]*The Times* (July 1, 1967).

[18]Now called *The Octopus*.

[19]Jon Ruddy, *MacLean's Magazine* (January, 1969), pp. 35-40.

[20]*The Times* (July 24, 1967), p. 5.

[21]*The Lancet* (November 9, 1963).

[22]George Brimmell, "U.S. drug chief stands firm on defence of marijuana," *Ottawa Citizen* (Oct. 26, 1967).

[23]"Pot Possession should be legal, psychologist says," *Globe and Mail* (March 5, 1968).

[24]G. Joseph Tauro, Chief Justice of the Superior Court of Massachusetts, Judgment on the appeal of J. D. Leis and Ivan Weiss, entered December 19, 1964. (typescript copy)

[25]Rick Mackie, "Law changes needed to prevent criminal empires," *Ottawa Citizen* (Oct. 6, 1967).

[26]"B.C. medical group rejects marijuana sale plan," *Globe and Mail* (Oct. 13, 1967).

[27]J. Robertson Unwin, "Illicit Drug Use Among Canadian Youth" (Part II), *Canadian Medical Association Journal*, vol. 98 (March 2, 1968), pp. 449-54.

[28]Krista Maeots, "Making 'pot' possession a crime is 'starkly unjust': doctor," *Ottawa Citizen* (Nov. 8, 1968).

[29]*Marihuana and its Effects: an Assessment of Current Knowledge*, A statement from the office of the Executive Director, Addiction Research Foundation of Ontario, *Addictions*, vol. 15, no. 1 (Spring, 1968), pp. 1-7.

[30]See, for example: "Psychologist says drug possession penalty too high," *Globe and Mail* (Nov. 30, 1967); Leone Kirkwood, "Half of pot users need aid, doctors tell health body," *Globe and Mail* (Sept. 28, 1968); "Marijuana penalties too severe, addiction centre director says," *Globe and Mail* (April 17, 1969).

[31]"Still working in the dark," *Globe and Mail* (April 18, 1969).

[32]John Howard Society of Ontario, Brief to the Hon. J. N. Turner, Minister of Justice, "Sanctions on Marihuana" (July 8, 1968), 9 pp.

[33]Geoffrey Stevens, "Bill would lighten drug use penalty," *Globe and Mail* (Oct. 18, 1968).

[34]17 Elizabeth II (1968) Senate of Canada, Bill S-15.

[35]Bob Cohen, "Drugs Worry Munro," *Ottawa Citizen* (Dec. 6, 1968).

[36]17-18 Elizabeth II (1969), c. 41, s. 12.

[37]"Change in Drug Act may put marijuana in different class," *Globe and Mail* (Dec. 20, 1968).

[38]Robert Fulford in *Saturday Night* (May, 1969), p. 17.

The Hallucinogenic Experience

One scarcely knows where to begin in describing LSD and what it does. The subject is curiously formless, maddeningly elusive, and congenitally unsuited to the traditional type of rational prose analysis that we have come to think of as being 'scientific'. It is almost impossible to speak meaningfully about the LSD-type experience without recourse to the language of poetry or to the shapes and colors of the visual understanding. Those who return to the mundane world after experiencing a mystical religious vision or a drug-induced ecstatic state or a psychotic trip into madness are notoriously unable to communicate their experience to those who have remained behind. They find themselves helplessly inarticulate, trying to express through words an understanding that loses its meaning and uniqueness the very moment it is put into words. If they give up and decide to keep their vision silently intact, they are accused of obscurantism and evasion. If by Herculean effort they manage to embody something of the experience in verbal form, they cannot fail at the same time to be conscious of how much they have lost. Imagine the difficulties of describing colors to one who is blind or to one who sees only in blacks and whites. Or sound to one who is deaf. Or imagine trying to translate music into prose.

These then are the difficulties. Anyone who tries to write about LSD without an understanding of this dimension of the problem is like a bird preparing to fly with only one wing. But if we must recognize the limits of 'rational' analysis, we must also recognize the dangers of throwing over rational analysis altogether, à la Timothy Leary, and lapsing into that state of mental incoherence in which 'blowing the mind' becomes all too literal a process. Even Dr. Leary feels constrained to write books in which some approximation of linear reasoning is utilized to bring across his message of non-linear enlightenment, just as Marshall McLuhan's celebration of the triumph of the electronic media has been largely carried out through the supposedly deposed print medium. Moreover the attempts that have been made to mix visual with printed information have not been, on the whole, very satisfactory in lighting up previously unknown areas of the mind. They quickly become stereotyped and the senses dulled to their meaning.[1]

This points to a further difficulty in writing about LSD – the incredible rapidity with which new concepts arising out of the discovery and use of LSD have been swallowed, denatured, regurgitated, packaged, and sold on the mass market by the commercial interests. In 1957 Dr. Humphry Osmond coined the word *psychedelic* to describe the particular "mind-manifesting" experience induced by LSD and similar hallucinogenic drugs.[2] A decade later the word was still largely a piece of scientific jargon. Then in 1967 the great LSD scare and the hippie cult became staples of the popular media. Today the word *psychedelic* has been so devalued as to be virtually meaningless. *Psychedelic* now refers to a pattern on a shirt in the bargain-basement of a department store or to the vulgar decorations set up by middle-aged swingers trying to hold a 'with-it' party.

The capitalist Saturn has an enormous capacity for eating his children. *Sic transit gloria.* Already the psychedelic cultists have a hopelessly *passé* look about them, like yesterday's newspapers or yesterday's pop singers. Those who make it their business to cling desperately to the crest of every popular wave have now abandoned the LSD scene and thereby declared it unfashionable, which is surely the gravest sin in the contemporary religion of *Now!* Nevertheless, only the most dedicated seekers after ephemera – those whom Edmund Burke memorably dismissed as the "flies of a summer" – need be deterred by the apparent unfashionableness of the topic, for if the reader is willing to jettison a good deal of intellectual garbage, whether from the underground or the above ground press, it may be found that after the waves have passed there still remains a good deal beneath the surface. Moreover, it is not LSD itself that is important, but the type of experience that LSD helped to bring before the public consciousness. We may kill the bearer of bad news (or what we think is bad news) but such an act does not change the message itself. In this case a judicious combination of commercial exploitation and political repression may succeed in doing in the messenger, but this fact in itself may not ultimately mean very much. The reaction of society in the face of such a message may mean far more.

Let us start at the beginning – or more precisely the modern beginning, for the use of hallucinogenic plants has been part of human culture for many millennia. In 1938 in the Sandoz Research Laboratories in Basle, Switzerland, d-lysergic acid diethylamide (LSD-25) was synthesized. At first the peculiar properties of the new drug were not known, but in 1943 Dr. Albert Hofmann, one of the two original discoverers of the substance, was working with LSD in the laboratory when he began to feel a "very peculiar restlessness". Returning home, he lay in bed and experienced what he interpreted to be "a not unpleasant state of drunkenness" during which he saw "phantastic images of an extraordinary plasticity . . . associated with an intense kaleidoscopic play of colours." Later, Dr. Hofmann, after deciding that he must have accidentally absorbed some of the new chemical, deliberately ingested 250 micrograms as an experiment. This time the experience was much more intense, and driving a bicycle from the laboratory to his home he became subject to serious perceptual distortion, such as the delusion that his bicycle was standing still. Terrified that he was becoming psychotic, he began interpreting negatively all that he saw. Faces turned into lurid masks. His tongue became metallic. He was standing outside himself, watching as he raved and shrieked. The next day he was wholly recovered, and what was later to become a vast volume of research on LSD was begun.[3]

Chemically, LSD is a partially-synthetic compound: lysergic acid is a natural product of the ergot fungus known as *Claviceps purpurea*, found on rye and other plants. Diethylamide is a synthetic related to ergonovine which is used medically as a uterine stimulant.[4] LSD is one of the most potent chemicals yet discovered insofar as immediately observable effects on man are concerned. It is thousands of times more potent than mescaline, which is itself a powerful hallucinogenic. One ounce contains enough average doses (100 micrograms or 1/10,000 gram) to send the entire population of Ottawa into a temporary state of drug-induced ecstasy or insanity, as the case may be. Theoretically, a briefcase filled with the drug could have the potential for incapacitating the entire country – a rather abstract and unrealistic fancy that has nevertheless led to some garish theorizing about LSD warfare. There is no question, however, about LSD's incredible potency, which becomes all the more amazing when it is considered that of the tiny amount normally ingested, at most only about one per cent is found in the brain. The bulk goes into the intestines, liver, and kidneys. What is more, in the forty-five minute period before the psychological effects usually begin, all LSD disappears from the brain. In effect, somewhat less than four million molecules of LSD come in contact with some ten billion brain cells for a few minutes. Yet this fleeting and seemingly superficial contact is sufficient to cause the most profound results. Possibly, the LSD itself must set off a chain of metabolic processes that continue long after the chemical itself has disappeared.[5]

The question of how LSD affects the workings of the mind is an extremely involved and complex one, and there is by no means agreement on the part of scientists who are studying the phenomenon. By way of brief summary of some contemporary thought on this matter, we may put forward the following explanation: the human mind does not merely perceive external phenomena naively, but rather filters all perception through a pre-existing structure, which is itself the result of previous experience, and which not only shapes and defines the perceptions that enter it, but is itself shaped by these perceptions. This structure might be termed the *image* of the world outside the self that any functioning creature, as an information-gathering and information-organizing system, must possess in order to survive within the environment in which it finds itself.[6] The distinguished scientist and philosopher J. Bronowski has written of the "interlocked picture of the world" that the brain constructs. This picture is not a passive record, but is the symbolic expression of our activity in nature. "The picture is not the look of the world but our way of looking at it."[7]

With the introduction of the electron microscope into biological research, a revolution has occurred in the understanding of the functioning of the brain. This in turn casts a good deal of light upon the precise impact of LSD on the brain's workings. The brain is composed of some ten billion nerve cells or *neurons*, linked together by a complex system of multichannel inputs and outputs. Information is transferred from neuron to neuron through contact points known as *synapses*, of which there may be up to 50,000 or more for each neuron.[8] This transfer is accomplished generally by means of a chemical transmitter that diffuses across the gap between synapses, and causes excitation of the receptor upon making contact. There are a number of such chemical transmitters; one of them is *serotonin*. One of the unique characteristics of LSD is that it powerfully inhibits serotonin.[9] It has been suggested that LSD may in fact decrease serotonin turnover by depressing the firing rate of neurons containing serotonin.[10]

To return to our original statement concerning the way in which the mind constructs a filter through which all perceptions must pass, it seems entirely possible that LSD tends to weaken, or to make more porous, the mind's filter. In effect the net (or 'reticular system' as it is more precisely known) that we set up to sort out what our experience has told us is relevant, and what is irrelevant, sensory data, is shredded by the powerful impact of LSD, and through the newly created holes a vast and uncontrolled amount of sensory data pours directly into the consciousness. If the synapses can be seen as the decision-points of the nervous system, then LSD puts the mind's defences in a state of disarray. As one neurophysiologist has written:

It is now an established principle of neurophysiology that complex control systems are continuously in operation in shaping, blocking or facilitating one or another channel of sensory information, and that this regulation of sensory input to the brain is variable under different conditions of sleep and wakefulness. Such mechanisms for controlling afferent input not only permit focussing of attention to a particular task or motor event, but also protect the brain from the cacaphonous interplay of the varied meaningless signals that continually bombard sensory receptors. Recent neurophysiological investigations indicate that much of the control of sensory input to the brain is regulated by projection pathways from nonspecific 'reticular systems' to primary sensory neurons in the spinal cord and brain stem. Little imagination is required to envision the consequences of disturbances initiated by LSD in these 'reticular systems'. . . . It is within these complex brain-stem networks that much of the synaptic business of integrating incoming and outgoing information is transacted, and it is here that LSD is most likely to cause profound physiological disturbances through its synaptic actions.[11]

If LSD simply played tricks with the individual's perceptions it might be thought a mild curiosity, but its effects are of deep significance not only for the individual but for civilization as a whole. The mental filter or net that LSD attacks is not merely a product of the individual's personal experience but is the cumulative result of the entire learning and socialization process to which every society by necessity subjects its members. No individual could continue to function if every contemplated action had to be thought out afresh each time – for example, nobody could live for long if they had to consciously *will* each breath, and make a specific decision on each heart beat. Similarly it is doubtful that a society, even a society in the throes of a political and social revolution, could long survive if a certain modicum of behavioral predictability could not be maintained in social relationships. People brought up in the same society tend to *see* things in roughly similar ways: individual perspectives are integrated to the extent that the mental filters of individuals are evolved and structured within the same social environment. But if we remember Bronowski's comment that "the picture is not the look of the world but our way of looking at it,"[12] we can quickly recognize that the way in which the individual member of any society structures his picture of the world is certain to be a partial and culturally limited *point of view* of a reality that is too complex to be wholly comprehended by any one person, just as a conventional 'picture' in the sense of a work of art, is in essence the interpretation of an individual perspective on reality, the meaning of which can be communicated to others to the extent that others either share the artist's perspective or can be brought to discover that perspective. LSD, then, is a *revolutionary* weapon that strikes, although only temporarily, at the deepest roots of a society's conservative foundations, at those aspects of the social definition of reality that have been internalized by individuals and have become so much a part of the individual's very structure of thought that he is no longer consciously aware of them. In 1958 a Czech doctor stated that "LSD inhibits conditioned reflexes". As poet Allen Ginsberg comments, "this single phrase, for rational men, might be the key to the whole Gnostic mystery of LSD."[13]

Imagine yourself standing along the shoreline of a vast ocean. You have walked along this shoreline many times before, vaguely conscious of the incomprehensible vastness of the ocean, knowing in an abstract sort of way that it is so many miles deep and so wide but not really grasping the meaning of figures that so greatly exceed the human scale. Perhaps when you were a child you once sat on the shore and *thought* about the sea, and perhaps it frightened you and so you thought no more about it. As you grew older and, as you thought, wiser, you no longer were even aware in your day-today life of what lay beyond the shore. You knew that the tide would rise just so far and no further and that the boundaries of your world were thus clearly and precisely defined.

Then one day the tide does not stop where it is supposed to stop, but continues to rise higher and higher. Like King Canute you order the waves back: "This is not proper . . . this is not rational . . . this is not the way the world is." But you have to retreat, and as you run you can no longer recognize the boundary between land and not-land, and then you realize that when that boundary disappears you begin to wonder what will happen to the boundaries of your own self, to the shoreline of the you and the not-you. You are afraid, more afraid than you have ever been before.

And now the great ocean rises beyond your worst nightmares. You throw up dykes of sand, which vanish with each new crest. You climb on to the tops of cliffs, but still the tide comes on. Just at the moment when you are most terrified, you begin to *see*, with blinding clarity, each luminous drop of water as a separate world, and the ocean itself as the whole universe in its infinite vastness, each drop of water a glittering star, a blazing sun, a soul, a flower, a word, an eye, a god, all these things at once and with an unbearable intensity from which you must desperately try to flee. With the same terrible clarity you recognize that your last defences are down and the cosmic ocean is at the last shoreline, between yourself and the outside. The dyke of sanity is breached, and Death is a great wave, as vast as all of space, and moving with the inexorable rhythm of time itself. Then from somewhere, from another world, comes a voice that urges you to surrender yourself to the wave, to give yourself up to death. Who after all are *you* amid this ocean? All that divides you from the outside world is washed away.

There is nothing left. You surrender, and the oceanic cosmos scatters your cells and molecules like so many grains of sand. *You* have died. But there is another *you* watching your own death. And this second self sees the joyous truth, that death is liberation, that 'death' is a beautiful blue tide, iridescent in the sunlight, and that the miserable inward being known as the self was only an accidental conjunction of particles that for a brief moment amid eternity became self-conscious, but which have now rejoined the great tide of life. Death is not death at all, but a necessary stage before rebirth – a dissolution of false personal boundaries in the laughing solvent of a deeper consciousness. You are part of the ocean, you *are* the ocean.

And now you rediscover the world. But it is no longer the same world to which you had grown accustomed. You have become a child once more, you are Adam or Eve awaking in the garden for the first time, you are a wandering poet of the thirteenth century seeing the new springtime of the world after the long centuries of darkness. There is a sense of wonder to everything. What was yesterday a mere commonplace is now a multi-faceted jewel. You are handed an apple and it has become a living creature, whose delicate and infinitely complex *apple-ness* is as important as the largest star in the universe. Someone smiles and the smile is a warm yellow sound, as clear and as perfect as a tinkling cymbal in the stillness of the afternoon. You hear a bird sing, and its song is a shimmering green raindrop falling on your inward sea, and you know that the gentle ripples from that drop will go on and on, all the days of your life.

This is one way it can happen. Unfortunately it is not the only way. The mind has many doors, many strange passageways, and rooms stranger yet. At the beginning it is a maze of mirror-lined routes, each reflecting another. It is possible to take the wrong turn. Some do.

There are people who have been wrecked by LSD or similar drugs. Somewhere a wrong turn has been made, and what could be a joyous revelation has become instead a grisly prison of the mind, a Hell without exit or hope. It has been reported that in the United States there is a young man who believes himself to be an orange. Since there is no way to reach him, there seems little hope that he will be anything but an orange for the rest of his life. Less spectacularly, one can sometimes see the toll of LSD in the eyes of young teenagers, bewildered, frightened, and curiously empty. Statistics on the incidence of good and bad trips are notoriously unreliable: very much depends on the source one consults. There does, however, seem to be some solid evidence that LSD has become statistically more dangerous over the past few years, in the sense that a greater proportion of bad trips have been coming to the attention of medical authorities. Of course it may be that with the greater familiarity of the medical profession with LSD, more psychoses have been identified with the use of the drug, but it is also likely that in the past few years LSD has increasingly fallen into the hands of those least able to handle its effects. We will return to this problem later, but first we must attempt to deal with a difficult question: why does LSD affect different people in radically different ways?

The ocean we pictured is a visual metaphor for one of the characteristic features of the LSD experience: the overwhelming flood of unclassified sensory data that pours past the mind's synaptic defence-points. It is in fact not uncommon for people to 'see' this process in the image of an oceanic tide. Some may see it as a wind that blows through them as if they were not real. Others may experience quite different images. One person reported to me that he hung by his fingers to a precipice overhanging an infinite abyss for a thousand years. When at last he could hold on no longer, he let his fingers open, and in a moment of enlightenment discovered that he had been hanging on to his own hair. Others, especially those who have already had a similar experience before, may not feel the perceptual flood to be a threat but may instead simply float along with it. Whatever the images involved, it is a characteristic of the LSD experience that there is in some sense a 'death', of the ego, of the self, of the cultural, social, and psychological identities that we spend a lifetime constructing. Such a death is necessary if rebirth is to follow. A newer and deeper consciousness can only rise, phoenix-like, on the ashes of the old. Of course, not everyone achieves rebirth. That is the problem.

Sidney Cohen suggests the following model of a 'good' experience.

Consider a man who had been living alone all his life in a private emotional fortress, busily engaged in deepening the moats and strengthening the parapets. Despite the prodigious defences he still feels unprotected and insecure. Furthermore, the walls are now so high that he has separated himself from people. He can only shout to them from the battlements and cannot quite make out what they are shouting back, but the sounds are unfriendly. One day a tremendous storm destroys his stronghold. He is defenceless. To his great surprise he is not demolished or even attacked. People seem friendly. What had he feared? His own hostility? Why was he never loved? Was it those impregnable walls? Maybe it would be better to trust and rejoin the human race than retreat behind the barriers again.[14]

In Freudian terms we might see the mighty inward struggle as a contest between the *Superego* and the *Id*, in which both aspects become concretized in some form which has mythic roots in the individual's consciousness.[15] This perspective accommodates one of the more peculiar phenomena associated with LSD, the persistence of an observing self at the same time as the self is in the act of dying. The quality of being both inside and outside oneself at the same time is an extremely difficult situation for anyone to conceptualize in their own minds if they have not experienced it personally. But with LSD it can become sometimes a very real, concrete experience. A subject may even report exact measurements of the extent of his personality-dissociation: "I am now one quarter of an inch outside myself," or "my body now has two heads and I am looking at my own face." Sometimes the dissociation will become very pronounced and a person may watch himself from a great distance. So it is that one can become a guest at one's own funeral, and a midwife to one's own birth. This may have a good deal of psychotherapeutic value since the almost literal 'detachment' of the self can ease the flood of repressed memories in a situation that would otherwise be unbearable.

One of the first things a newborn child must learn is the boundary between itself and the outside world. Gradually through trial and error it learns to distinguish the point where it stops and the environment begins. LSD puts a grown person back into the position of the baby. Since much of the definition of the self may be false or illusory or even destructive, such a reversion can be useful to the individual as a means of understanding what he is and, more importantly, what he can become. Psychotherapeutically, LSD-induced *regression* may be a valuable tool inasmuch as the patient's early history can be relived in a very concrete fashion. One psychoanalyst who is engaged in a long-term study of the use of LSD in psychotherapy has recently stated that "ten years of clinical work with LSD have led me to think that regression is the key to whatever virtue there is in LSD-facilitated psychotherapy. It is also the main source of whatever psychological damage is done by LSD."[16] It may also help to explain much of the popularity of LSD: to see the world once again through the eyes of a child can be a very beautiful experience. It is also a particularly sought-after gift in an age in which there is so much revulsion against the world that 'adults' have made and so much searching for what appears to be our lost innocence.

Other phenomena associated with LSD that should be mentioned in passing are *synaesthesia* and *eidetic conceptualization*. Both can occur naturally, but they are sufficiently rare to require explanation. Synesthesia is the expression of one sensory input in terms of another. That is to say, one sees a sound, or hears a taste. The sudden ringing of a telephone during an LSD session may appear to the subject as a jagged purple flash before his eyes. The explanation would seem to be that the individual is subjected to sensory overload and when too much information pours into one channel, some may spill out into another. If we are struck on the head and the pain briefly flares up above our capacity to fully feel it, we may "see stars": which is simply a sensory overload spilling out into the visual channel. People who value the LSD experience often point to the synaesthetic phenomenon as a means of deepening one's perception of, say, music, by allowing one to appreciate it visually as well as by ear. Whether such enhanced appreciation is actual or merely apparent is a problem that we cannot deal with here, but it could be pointed out now that the trend in recent years toward mixed-media forms in art is an attempt to build the synaesthetic dimension into the performance itself, presumably on the assumption that it represents a deeper level of artistic consciousness.

Eidetic conceptualization refers to the tendency of the mind under LSD to give concrete, usually visual, embodiment to abstract ideas. Such embodiment often takes the form of elaborate mythic dramas. Indeed the eidetic content of the LSD experience might suggest a more precise name than that of *hallucinogenic*, which has the sense of giving hallucinations, or mere optical illusions. In fact, real but undefined personal problems can take the form of people or animals or things, and, caught up in what appears to the individual to be a very real and living situation, an allegorical or metaphorical drama unfolds, within which the individual may discover a deeper understanding of the processes at work within himself. Fears and anxieties may become dragons or demons or dwarfs. Greek myths, Gothic fairy tales, far-flung science fiction dramas, primitive rituals, a reliving of eons of evolutionary development, re-enactments of historical events — all these may serve as the eidetic conceptualizations of inner conflicts, fears, and desires. Sometimes a truly cosmological scale is achieved as God wars with Satan for mastery of the universe, or the individual becomes a tiny speck of consciousness floating in the great void, seeing the genesis and death of whole universes. The psychological connection between this eidetic phenomenon and the place of dreams in psychotherapy is immediately obvious. The LSD experience may, however, be much more powerful with much greater conscious impact on the subject. For that very reason, it presents a greater opportunity, and a greater danger.

It is yet another typical aspect of the LSD experience that external objects, even those that we normally classify as being inanimate, will appear as sentient beings. It is not at all uncommon for someone to see an orange or a grape or even a wine glass or a garbage tin as a living, breathing, palpitating creature. In part this is a visual trick that, under conditions of sensory overload, makes the outlines of objects seem to waver. But there is more to it than this. We normally classify objects in a relational or in a functional sense. That is to say, an orange exists to be eaten or a garbage tin exists to hold garbage. A wine glass may be appreciated as much for its graceful beauty as for its usefulness in holding wine, but even here its 'function' is to please the human eye. LSD does a very interesting thing, however: one no longer perceives objects within a pre-existing framework of meaning; instead one simply perceives, without a structure of meaning to guide the interpretation of the sensory data. The result is that objects tend to be seen in terms only of themselves. An orange no longer has to fulfill some externally-imposed function, it rather expresses its own *orangeness*. A chair need not exist *for* something else, it simply *is*. It constitutes, in other words, what Kant called the *Ding an Sich*, the thing-in-itself.

All this may seem harmless enough but in some strange and undefined manner it seems to represent a concept that is deeply subversive of the whole Western attitude toward the natural world as a realm for conquest and domination, as inert material to be shaped to man's will and purpose. In the Christian genesis, God gave to Adam the right to *name* all the creatures of the earth and by this symbolic act man gained mastery over the rest of nature. When the symbolic meaning of language is inhibited or disordered, as with LSD, the non-human is liberated from human categories, and *things* are restored to their natural dignity and beauty. It is striking how often this insight is offered as an example of the higher level of consciousness said to be achieved by drug-induced states. Perceived with extreme intensity, unfettered by externally imposed meanings, objects are seen to possess a beautiful, sometimes terrifying power – to shine forth with an 'inner light'.

As with marijuana and hashish, LSD often tends to distort the perception of time and space. It is not uncommon for an LSD subject to crouch down for fear of striking his head on a ceiling, even though the ceiling may in fact be many feet above his head. More interesting perhaps are the time effects, which may vary from minor confusions concerning the passage of a few minutes to the firmly implanted conviction that months, even years, have elapsed during a period that is objectively measured in a handful of hours. It might appear on the surface that this is merely another perceptual trick, either amusing or dangerous depending on the circumstances, but once again there is more than meets the eye. We too often forget that our measurements of time and space have nothing whatever to do with objective reality but are instead constructions of our own minds. While there may be real electrons and real protons, there are no 'real' inches or 'real' minutes. The latter are human categories imposed on reality that, despite their obvious usefulness, can also be misleading or inadequate. Turkish villagers used to a day-long journey to Ankara by foot were convinced that Istanbul was much closer because they reached it within only a few hours by train. In fact Istanbul was some three hundred miles farther, but the villagers measured distance by the time it took to travel – a perfectly logical method where a single means of transportation exists. A member of an African tribe that lived in extremely dense jungle was taken to a hill overlooking a wide valley. Observing some cattle far off in the distance he remarked with great astonishment that there should exist animals so tiny. Never having seen objects that were more than a few feet away he had developed no real concept of depth perception.

Such instances of man's own construction of the parameters of space and time are easy enough to point out with regard to so-called 'primitive' peoples. With regard to ourselves it is very much more difficult. Yet everyday language contains the dim recognition that objective time measurements may sometimes be less than adequate. We speak, for instance, of a "few short minutes," "long hours," or the "wee small hours of morning," and prissy grammarians may on occasion dismiss such usage as being illogical or contradictory. In fact it suggests a recognition of the importance of the subjective dimension in estimating time. Rather more spectacularly it is now recognized by scientists (post-Einstein) that if one were to set off on a space craft on a round trip to the nearest star, one would return after what would seem to be only a few years to find that centuries had elapsed on earth. What this points out is how technology alters not only the subjective but also the objective measurement of time and space. An important question is how adequate are our perceptual responses to a rapidly changing environment. As one urban planner has recently suggested:

... We have been too impressed by the machine, by the mass media of communication, and we imagine that the earth is shrinking. The earth is not shrinking, man is expanding. But this is an expansion of his senses, of his speed. In the small units of his living space and in his personal human relationships, man's scale remains what it has always been.[17]

To bring this discussion back to its starting point, we might point out that the space-time 'distortions' experienced with LSD may be no less distorted than what pass for objective measurements. Moreover the free play of the perceptual imagination may reveal space-time relationships which are not merely novel or amusing, but which may prove useful as well. There are apparently cases of architects whose creative processes have been 'unblocked' through the insight that an LSD experience offered in the face of a previously insoluble problem of spatial relationships. A concrete example of this is a clinic in Weyburn, Saskatchewan.

In a period of rapid and seemingly chaotic change anything such as LSD that inhibits conditioned responses and disorganizes learned patterns of behavior *may* have creative potential. New perceptual relationships may be perceived that 'click' with a new reality. The dangers, of course, are just as obvious. Einstein suggested that space and time

considered logically ... are free creations of the human intelligence, tools of thought, which are to serve the purpose of bringing experiences into relation with each other, so that in this way they can be better surveyed. The attempt to become conscious of the empirical sources of these fundamental concepts should show to what extent we are actually bound to these concepts. In this way we become aware of our freedom, of which, in case of necessity, it is always a difficult matter to make sensible use.[18]

Above and beyond all these secondary characteristics of the LSD experience that we have been describing, at the very heart of the transcendental or 'ecstatic' state of drug-induced consciousness lies a feeling of the great cosmic unity of life, a mystical level of understanding that is difficult, if not impossible, to render in words. It is fair to suggest that what many LSD users take to be mystical experiences are hardly worthy of the name, but the difficulty in separating the genuine from the merely superficial is compounded by the inability to communicate an essentially non-verbal experience into the framework of language. Perhaps the only objective criterion we can apply is to test whether any observable changes in behavior follow what purport to be mystical experiences. In this sense much of the 'love' mythology surrounding the hippie cult can be exposed as ersatz, inasmuch as it is high on verbal protestations but rather lower on genuine love-oriented behavior. A particularly striking example of how silly and misleading the LSD experience can appear is afforded by a subject of Masters and Houston who claimed that with LSD she had achieved a "Christ-like love of all beings". Unfortunately she was asked to elaborate during the experience itself. The following verbal diarrhoea ensued.

Negroes and little fishes, lampshades and vinegar. These I love. Coats and hats and three-ring pretzels. Radios and Russians, bobolinks and tree sap, medicine chests and Freud and the green line down the centre of the street on St. Patrick's Day, these I love. These I cherish. My old blue sweater and the Cherokees. Pots and pans and cold cream and books and stores and the dear little moron on ——— Street who sells the comic books. Hair spray and Buddha and Krishna Menon. My love overfloweth to all. My nephew and mushrooms. Red cars, red caps, porters, Martin Luther King, Armenians, Jews, Incas and John O'Hara. Love. Love. Love. Big yellow chrysanthemums and the sun and pancakes and Disneyland and Vermont and cinnamon and Alexander the Great. The UN and aluminum foil and apple cider and cigars. Clark Gable, Tony Curtis and salamanders, crochet, the aurora borealis and dimples, mustard plasters and even Mayor Wagner. I am just bursting with joy, with love. I want to give . . . Give to all . . . Give . . . My Love . . . To . . . All . . .[19]

And so on. And on. And on. And on.

Masters and Houston further note that there was "no subsequent observable change in her behavior to make the alleged love credible". In light of the above it is not surprising that William Burroughs has warned that prolonged use of LSD leads "in some cases to a crazed unwholesome benevolence, the old tripster smiling into your face sees all your thoughts loving and accepting you inside out."[20]

At the core of the LSD experience there may, however, sometimes be found a vision, at once profound, mystical, shattering, and ineffable. "If the doors of perception were cleansed," wrote William Blake, "everything will appear to man as it is, infinite." The doors of our perception are thickly encrusted so that the light of the Out There can scarcely penetrate, and what does penetrate is already shaped and structured so that it 'fits' the image we already possess of our environment. This is as it must be. The long evolutionary process through which life has struggled has involved the function of selecting adaptations that make the organism biologically viable. Part of this may be the progressive elimination from the consciousness of all sensory data that is inessential to the organism's need for survival. The complex differentiation of the human brain may thus be seen not as a superior receiver of data, but as a superior eliminator of data. After all, dogs can smell much better than we can, and can hear a wider range of sounds; some birds can see detail from much greater distances than we can. While I am sitting at my desk writing this paragraph I am unconsciously suppressing a vast amount of sensory data for the purpose of concentrating my conscious processes of thought on the *specific* matter at hand, just as the reader is suppressing a vast amount of data for the purpose of understanding what is written. It is utterly unnecessary for either of us to be constantly aware of the beating of our hearts or the minute differentiation of the colors of the sky, of the consistency of our breathing or the myriad sounds occurring simultaneously inside and outside ourselves. In fact if we were constantly aware of all these things we would never be able to marshall our faculties for any specific task. But if we have gained a superior flexibility and adaptability through the brain's power of selectively eliminating information, we have also lost something. We are now able to perceive with vast detail and with great subtlety the extent of our *separation* from the outside world. We are much less able to understand the extent to which we are a *part* of that world.

In the Western world this antithesis of the Self and the Outside has been symbolized in the contrast between the Mind and the Body, or the Spirit and the Flesh, which are in turn closely related to the dualistic Christian theology of God and the Devil, Heaven and Hell, absolute Good and absolute Evil. It has been suggested many times that this dualism sets up a conflict within the individual that cannot be resolved. After all, we are both mind *and* body, one and inseparable, and any doctrine that teaches the one half to fear and mistrust the other half has rather obvious drawbacks. Modern science ironically enough owes its fundamental philosophical postulate to this same source of Christian dualism, transformed into the antithesis between what Descartes called the *res cogitans* and the *res extensa*, that is, between the sentient mind and the natural world that the mind can observe and explain without in any way interfering with its workings. Technology is simply the application of power to this division, the concept that man the thinker can transform the material world for his own ends until eventually the mind entirely controls matter by means of the tools designed by the mind for that purpose. So the theory runs.

What is astonishing and exciting about the LSD experience is the twofold discovery that we have been operating mentally upon a very narrow and restricted level of consciousness, and that when one is able to transcend the everyday categories of thought, one can become aware that the dualistic image of the world is merely the product of one level of consciousness. More fundamental than apparent dualities is the Oneness of the universe, and into this unity the self is dissolved. This sense of wholeness is what Alan Watts found with LSD,[21] what Aldous Huxley found with mescalin,[22] what William James found with nitrous oxide[23] and, perhaps more importantly, what numerous saints, mystics, and ascetics have also found without the use of drugs. Eastern religions, especially Buddhism and Hinduism, have never held a dualistic view of the world and it is thus not surprising that the attempts of the Western mind to grapple with this concept have often taken on Eastern trappings. Leary and Alpert, for instance, attempt to fit the LSD experience into the form set out in the *Tibetan Book of the Dead*.[24] The oriental trappings are merely secondary, perhaps largely adventitious. What is important is the vision itself. It is this that a Canadian psychiatrist at the turn of the century called "Cosmic Consciousness".[25]

William James experimented with nitrous oxide (laughing gas) with results very relevant to those we are discussing here.

One conclusion was forced upon my mind . . . and my impression of its truth has ever since remained unshaken. It is that our normal waking consciousness as we call it, is but one special type of consciousness, whilst all about it, parted from it by the filmiest of screens, there lie potential forms of consciousness entirely different . . . No account of the universe in its totality can be final which leaves these other forms of consciousness quite disregarded . . . they forbid a premature closing of our accounts with reality. Looking back on my own experiences, they all converge towards a kind of insight to which I cannot help ascribing some metaphysical significance. The keynote of it is invariably a reconciliation. It is as if the opposite of the world, whose contradictoriness and conflict make all our difficulties and troubles, were melted into unity. Not only do they, as contrasted species, belong to one and the same genus, but *one of the species, the nobler and better one, is itself the genus, and so soaks up and obsorbs its opposite into itself.* This is a dark saying, I know, when thus expressed in terms of common logic, but I cannot wholly escape from its authority .... Those who have ears to hear, let them hear; to me the living sense of its reality only comes in the artificial mystic state of mind.[26]

To appreciate this statement fully, it should be remembered that James was one of the founders of the American school of pragmatism in philosophy and in no way the sort of man ready to accept mystical ideas at face value. To take another example, Aldous Huxley suggested from the experience of his mescalin experiment: "In the final stage of ego-lessness there is an 'obscure knowledge' that All is in all – that All is actually each. This is as near, I take it, as a finite mind can ever come to 'perceiving everything that is happening everywhere in the universe'."[27] George Harrison says it more simply in one of his songs: "Life flows on, within you and without you".

I recall very vividly a personal experience that perhaps borders, although only slightly, on the above accounts. It was very early spring and all day fresh snow had been falling – inordinately large, glittering, extremely beautiful snowflakes. In the evening, the relatively warm temperature caused a thick white mist to form. I went for a long walk across wide, empty country fields. The mist became thicker and soon there were no sounds whatever, only the whiteness and the silence. But gradually stars began to appear from above, glinting through the mist, and these were reflected in the sparkling snowflakes below. Soon it became impossible to tell which were stars and which snowflakes. At this point a very peculiar thing happened – I lost all sense of which direction was up and which down, or more precisely, the problem ceased to have any meaning in much the same way that it ceases to have meaning to an astronaut outside the earth's gravitational field. The latter analogy is a helpful one, for I now felt as if I were floating amid the stars. But in contrast to the black, foreboding emptiness of space, that terrible infinity of nothingness that so haunts our already frightened imagination in what we call the Space Age, this cosmos that I was drifting through was *white* space, out of which all the lonely vastness had been expelled. Space was no longer an absence, but a presence. Just as white is a reflection of all the colors of the spectrum, so the universe had become a carnival of life, a joyous medley of all that moves, breathes, pulses, grows and changes. I was no longer adrift amid meaningless mathematical abstractions, nor amid discrete, alienated entities turned inward upon themselves, planets and people relentlessly following the ironclad physical laws of nature in eternal solitude. I had once thought this way, but now I saw – or better, I felt – that the universe was a *biological* wholeness, and that space was an amniotic fluid. There was no longer any question of distances; the universe was a seamless simultaneity of living matter.

The moment passed very quickly. A critical observer might well ask what such an experience proves. All I can say is that it impressed itself upon me as something very radically out of the ordinary, as a revelation or discovery of a truth that has always been there and always will be there. Moreover it opened up a perspective on life that had been largely closed to me before. The snow, the mist, and other accidental climatic factors had triggered a set of reactions that altered my consciousness – and what I had seen and felt at this different level of consciousness was every bit as 'real' and memorable as that which one sees and feels when visiting a strange country.

When someone takes a drug such as LSD they are simply registering a specific intent to undertake a change in consciousness, to travel to another country of the mind. It is important to make clear the distinction between the drug and the drug experience, but it is also important to remember their relationship. It is not logical to say that the experience is legitimate, even valuable, but that taking a drug in order to achieve such an experience is immoral. If there is a locked room you want to enter you will need a key, but once the door is opened the key's usefulness has ended. Nor is it logical to deny the value of such experiences because they were brought about through the use of a drug. Next to my desk as I write I have a photograph of a rock, a few feet in diameter, resting on a gravelly slope. This rock was not photographed by a human being nor does it exist anywhere on the earth. In fact it lies on the surface of the Moon, where, at the moment this is being written, no human has yet trod. Yet I can 'see' this moon rock almost as clearly as an earth rock a few feet away. Does the 'artificial' means whereby this photograph was taken impair its value? Is it any the less truthful an image than that of the naked eye, which can discern only the most general geological features on the moon's face? When explicitly posed the questions appear absurd, but no less absurd than similar questions directed against the use of psychedelic chemicals as cleansers of the doors of perception. Space craft, cameras, and consciousness-altering chemicals are all means of extending our senses.

The absurdity of this point of view is further driven home when one examines the basis of many so-called 'natural' mystical experiences. It was no accident that so many Christian mystics were ascetics. It has now been clearly established that sensory deprivation can bring about much the same state of mind as sensory overload. Both reduce the efficiency of the brain's sorting mechanisms. Aldous Huxley has aptly summarized what we now understand of the ascetic's methods in the light of modern knowledge.

... it is a matter of historical record that most contemplatives worked systematically to modify their body chemistry, with a view to operating the internal conditions favorable to spiritual insight. When they were not starving themselves into low blood sugar and a vitamin deficiency, or beating themselves into intoxication by histamine, adrenaline, and decomposed protein, they were cultivating insomnia and praying for long periods in uncomfortable positions, in order to create the psycho-physical symptoms of stress. In the intervals they sang interminable psalms, thus increasing the amount of carbon dioxide in the lungs and blood-stream, or, if they were Orientals, they did breathing exercises to accomplish the same purpose. Today we know how to lower the efficiency of the cerebral reducing valve by direct chemical action, and without the risk of inflicting serious damage on the psycho-physical organism. For an aspiring mystic to revert, in the present state of knowledge, to prolonged fasting and self flagellation would be as senseless as it would be for an aspiring cook to behave like Charles Lamb's Chinaman, who burned down the house in order to roast a pig.[28]

Huxley also adds the important point that while artists, mystics, and visionaries ought to consult modern technical specialists, so too such specialists ought to consult artists, mystics, and visionaries who know what to do with the experiences thus made possible.

The point is not that religious mysticism loses its meaning when its chemical basis is revealed, any more than drug-induced experiences lose their value because of their immediate chemical cause. If we set aside the dualistic conception of the noble, abstract mind versus the degraded, sinful flesh and start over again with Marx's dictum that it is impossible to separate thought from matter that thinks, then we can see that the division between ideas and bio-chemistry of thought is as untenable as trying to separate the back of something from the front, or to separate up from down, or width from height: the one is meaningless without the other.

Earlier, when discussing what is known about the neurophysiological action of LSD, it was suggested that the chemical substance itself only serves to trigger a chain of metabolic processes, and that when the observable effects begin, the chemical has already left the brain. This is a very important point for it demonstrates in a striking manner that the drug itself is only a key. What happens when the door is opened is not in this sense *caused* by the key; the latter simply facilitates a process that has no intrinsic connection with the key at all. The door could be battered down, or another key could be fabricated, or one might find a way around the door. The key is merely a neutral tool.

This line of reasoning seems plausible and convincing. Yet when the opponents of gun-control legislation say that "guns don't kill; people kill" one feels that there is something amiss in the logic. Of course a gun does not kill anyone unless a human being pulls the trigger, but if the gun was not easily available the killing might not take place, since other methods are less efficient. While murderous desires may not depend on the existence of guns, nevertheless the more guns there are available the more likely it is that such desires will be translated into actual murders. Moreover it is at least arguable that the technological ease with which killing can be accomplished through the medium of a gun may in itself encourage the increasing acceptance of killing as a possible form of personal behavior. By this light it is not enough to say that technology is merely an extension of man; by facilitating the realization of all the possibilities inherent in the species, technology also extends the scope of the self-destructive possibilities. *Psychedelic* means *mind-manifesting*; psychedelic chemicals are technological means of bringing out some of the possibilities inherent in the mind. The chemical does not program a specific pattern of behavior. What happens during the experience itself is a product of the complex interaction between the sensory input and what is already in existence in the mind. But by facilitating the process of consciousness-alteration, LSD also enhances the destructive possibilities inherent in the mind. In 'manifesting' the mind, psychedelics do not specify what kind of mind, or what parts of the mind.

Throughout this book, great emphasis has been laid on the personality of drug users and the environment in which drugs are taken as determinants of the drug experience. Anything said in this regard about other drugs applies doubly for LSD and the other powerful hallucinogenics. It has been noted very often how a chance remark or an accidental occurrence early in an LSD session may set the tone for the entire experience. Any suggestion of fear or uneasiness, for example, may turn an acid trip into a nightmare of paranoia. A real or imagined feeling of hostility on the part of another person may turn the 'joyous cosmology' into a living hell of incipient psychosis. I have dwelt at some length upon the positive side of the hallucinogenic experience, not out of any wish to advertise its benefits, but to counteract what seems to be the prevalent current opinion of the media and of government, that LSD is not only bad, but utterly without value as well. This is far from the truth. But it would be equally dishonest to avoid the negative side. The hippie equivalent of the gun-control opponent might, and does say: "LSD does not make people mad; people make themselves mad." But he cannot have it both ways. If LSD can be justified as a technical aid to achieving new and valuable levels of consciousness, it is also a technical aid to going mad.

To counterpose the happy experiences we have described so far, we could put forward the case of another famous contemporary figure, that of Jean-Paul Sartre. In the 1930s Sartre, during a period of profound personal malaise, was given mescalin as an experimental subject. The psychiatrist made the mistake of warning Sartre that the experience might prove somewhat disagreeable. Prophecies of this sort tend to be self-fulfilling and after ingesting the drug, Sartre saw umbrellas turned into vultures, shoes into skeletons, and just out of the corner of his eye, crabs, octopuses, and 'grimacing things'. When Simone de Beauvoir telephoned the hospital to find out how the experiment was turning out, Sartre informed her that he was struggling with an octopus and that the octopus was having the better of it. He did, however, retain enough lucidity to blame the doctor's predictions for his condition. The symptoms disappeared, but then spontaneously recurred a few weeks later, when he became certain that he was being pursued by crabs. Sartre was terrified and believed himself to be entering a "chronic hallucinatory psychosis". Eventually convinced that the trouble was in his own failure to grapple with his personal problems, Sartre got past this dangerous stage in his psychological development but the mescalin experience was perhaps one of the more harrowing in his life.[29]

One of the 'lifelines', which is normally on hand during the LSD experience, is the knowledge that what is happening is the result of a drug. One part of the self is affected, but another part knows why it is affected. When this consciousness is not present, chaos may well result. Small children who have accidentally swallowed LSD have usually had ghastly experiences. First of all, they have no idea of what is going on, and secondly they have not yet had time in their young lives to build up a strong identity. The attack of LSD on the ego can thus be utterly devastating as there is nothing left to put the pieces back together. Similarly, were a person to be given LSD without his knowledge, the results would be predictably psychotic. In fact there is a well-documented case of a woman in New York city who, at an office party, was given a drink to which LSD had been added as a practical joke. Believing herself to have gone utterly insane, the unfortunate woman leaped to her death from a window.

If I might be allowed to relate another personal experience, I might perhaps cast some more light on the subtle gradations between a 'good' and a 'bad' experience. When I was a young boy I was given ether as part of a routine operation. At that time they simply put a mask over one's face and pumped the evil-smelling substance into one's nostrils. The immediate effect was one of extreme paranoia – as if the doctors were trying to kill you. After losing consciousness I suddenly found myself on a gigantic fiery wheel, which was moving with inexorable and sickening speed. Around the wheel there was only black nothingness. What was most astonishing was an overpowering sense of infinity, of unfathomable vastness, and of an almost blinding, larger-than-life vividness. With violent clarity I recognized that this was not like dreams, those flimsy, insubstantial will-o'-the-wisps. This was more real than reality itself. For a small boy to be cast into such a hell was doubly disastrous, for I was unable to recognize what was happening to me. I was utterly, abjectly terrified.

As this vast, nauseous wheel of fire dragged me relentlessly on its senseless journey I wanted only to get off. But there was nowhere to escape to. The wheel was everything. *This was it.* Eventually as the anaesthesia faded the words of some banal popular song of the time kept playing over and over in my head, "That's all there is, there isn't any more . . . ." The words were now malignant and leering. Happily I was able to put the whole matter into a small corner of my mind where it has stayed ever since as an unsettling memory.

At the time of this experience I knew nothing of the Hindu religion. It was thus with some astonishment that I learned years later of the Hindu concept of the great and terrible wheel of death and rebirth. One writer has suggested that the wheel is the separation of the mind from the world, the compulsion of the intellect to imagine that there is something else, other than the world. But *"there is only this world. There is nothing else."*[30] When one accepts this, one is set free from the wheel. That is all very well, but for a small boy such insight is not likely. Instead the experience was simply nightmarish. It was, in the fullest sense of the phrase, *too much*. Even now I could not contemplate re-entering that terrible world no matter how much I might learn from it. And yet what a thin line separates this nightmare from the joyous experience I recounted earlier. In both, the sense of the unity of all things was central. But the unity of an evil world is even worse than a fragmented evil. It all depends on the premise with which you begin.

For those who are at relative peace with themselves and with the world, the hallucinogenic experience will probably be a deeply moving and important event. For the average person, it *may* be – indeed if the environment is right and if a knowledgeable and understanding guide is in attendance, the chances are in favor of a 'good' experience. But for some, especially the psychologically disturbed, the apprehensive, and the very young, it might be the step that pushes them over the delicate borderline into overt insanity, that causes a long term derangement of the individual's capacity for adaptation and personal development. 'Mind-manifesting' or 'liberating the Id' as unqualified social programs are about as sensible as recommending that everybody 'do their thing'. It all depends upon what your 'thing' is. Hitler and Stalin did their things. Lyndon Johnson did his thing in Vietnam, and the Russians in Prague. To put it as bluntly as possible, not everybody's mind should be manifested; in fact many are best left alone. This is a hard saying, but it must be said. Timothy Leary will not say it, and to this extent he is a false, and dangerous, prophet.

We spoke earlier of religious mysticism as an analogy to the LSD trip. But at the other end of the spectrum is another analogy, that of schizophrenic psychosis. Research into the hallucinogenics first began as an attempt to induce a model psychosis. It now seems that the LSD experience is somewhat the same but also differs from the schizophrenic experience. One difference is obviously that the LSD subject *knows* that his unusual experiences are only temporary and drug-induced; to the schizophrenic, however, they are the ceaseless condition of life. Take, for example, the intensity with which objects are often viewed with LSD. This 'inner light' might seem beautiful or striking when it occurs for a few hours, but imagine what it would be like to live forever in a land where everything, every tiny detail, burns with what must come to seem like a fiendish intensity. One schizophrenic has described the world she inhabited as the "land of intolerable glare".[31] To get an idea of what this must mean, look at some of the paintings of the poor mad Van Gogh, with his landscapes of unbearable color and violence.

It now appears that in the light of research being undertaken into the chemical basis of schizophrenia, there may be an LSD-like substance secreted in the brain of the schizophrenic person. We cannot go into this point further except to suggest that the close similarity between the two ought to act as a warning light against an insouciant attitude toward hallucinogenic drugs.

And yet at a deeper level, it may be a mistake to draw a too-sharp antithesis between mystic visions on the one hand and insanity on the other. Indeed, one of the most compelling aspects of LSD experiments has been the light they have shed on how close the visionary and the schizophrenic worlds are in many aspects. Perhaps earlier ages – before 'mental health' became a civic duty akin to patriotism and right-thinking moral precepts, and before psychotherapy became a part of everyday life, when the madman and the holy man were often one and the same person – had a more instinctive understanding of the vast non-rational areas of human consciousness. To be a visionary or a mystic you must be a little mad, you must in fact be quite literally 'out of your mind' on a qualitatively different plane of consciousness from ordinary persons. The contemporary world may reluctantly admit this point, while at the same time ignoring the mystic's visions as being 'irrational' or 'unscientific' or 'not empirically verifiable'. But very few would admit the opposite, that to be mad, you must possess a vision not the property of ordinary mortals. We treat the 'mentally ill' as being mentally deficient or mentally incompetent, cripples in the game of life – as if the majority condition is synonymous with 'mental health' in some ultimate sense. This psychological totalitarianism is at last coming under fire from at least some quarters. The validity of referring to mental states as healthy or diseased by analogy to the condition of physical organisms has been strongly questioned on the basis that there is no single optimum mental state to be used as a model.[32] A Navaho Indian with cancer is pretty much in the same position as a white businessman with cancer. But the psychology and motivation considered necessary for the businessman's career might be considered maniacal by the Navaho, while the Navaho might be considered a hopeless case of psychological inadequacy by the businessman.

Some have gone further and suggested that our own society needs desperately to recapture some of the other modes of knowing, besides the narrowly rational and scientific. The French writer Michel Foucault has shown how the madman once had a certain voice in the conversation of mankind until the modern age drove him out of sight and into asylums. Foucault, if I understand him correctly, argues that the rational is only one side of human understanding, and that the non-rational – the mythic, visionary, emotional, intuitive, dreamlike elements of our being – has been suppressed and denied by modern scientific rationalism. The result is that the fruitful dialectic between the rational and the non-rational has broken down, and the rational element is without its proper stimulus, thus being forced to turn inward upon itself in an increasingly sterile and desperate search for meaning. Madness is not simply a degeneration of the mind but is a mode of knowing normally closed to the sane.[33] R. D. Laing, a radical psychoanalyst, has suggested that

We respect the voyager, the explorer, the climber, the space man. It makes far more sense to me as a valid project — indeed, as a desperately urgently required project for our time, to explore the inner space and time of consciousness. Perhaps this is one of the few things that still make sense in our historical context. We are so out of touch with this realm that many people can now argue seriously that it does not exist. It is very small wonder that it is perilous indeed to explore such a lost realm.[34]

The opportunities and the dangers are of one piece. No surgery is possible. Yet technological rationalism also claims its victims – in the rice-paddies of Vietnam, in the decaying and poisoned cities of North America, in the destruction of the natural environment. Beside these crimes, the dangers of the religious-schizophrenic-drug voyage seem miniscule. But how many bills have been introduced into Parliament to outlaw the possession of automobiles as being injurious to the health of those who use them as well as of those who only breathe the carbon monoxide with which they fill the air?

How can a society like our own accommodate the divine madness of voyaging inward? It certainly cannot do so if it remains itself unchanged. Here is where the problem arises, for while the system is normally willing to tolerate dissent so long as that dissent threatens no concrete change, all its forces of resistance are mobilized when the realization of dissenting views seems possible. The drug experience represents no direct political challenge to the system, but it does offer an alternative vision, a glimpse of that which technological society has erased from our consciousness, a sense of the older, the deeper, perhaps even the wiser, part of our senses. There is, then, the obscure sense that the drug experience represents a sort of pre-revolutionary consciousness, a weakening of that moral fibre that is the real sinew of the system, that it signifies the potential for a sort of General Strike of the internalized commitments of subjects to the State.[35]

Legislators who see anarchists and seditionists under every beard can however rest easily with regard to the actual drug cult as it has developed in North America, because it is so confused and chaotic that its only threat is to itself. It is interesting, however, to compare the contemporary hippie-drug movement with earlier historical parallels. Utopian and millenarian cults sprang up in the Middle Ages that attracted groups which in effect constituted surplus population with no settled social position – alienated intellectuals, lower clergy, and partially educated laymen.[36] The original Digger movement – not to be confused with contemporary hippie groups – tried to build, in seventeenth-century England, a community held together not by economic interests or by power but rather by the common relationship to God. The Anabaptists tried to unite their community around the direct and ecstatic confrontation with the divine.[37] So too there is today a surplus population, particularly of the young, which automation has rendered inessential. And the psychedelic cult is not dissimilar to earlier millenarian movements in its attempt to organize itself exclusively around a direct relationship with the infinite. Such movements may serve a useful purpose in bringing forward elements of human wisdom too easily forgotten by Western society. But they must by necessity be minor cults. Someone has to grow the food, and clean the streets and care for the sick.

But what of the chronic users of LSD? Does there exist the danger of a psychological dependency on the drug? Many people who have taken LSD and found it a valuable experience have no interest in taking it again. One of Sidney Cohen's subjects, who in fact had the most blissful response of all, was offered another dose and refused: "I've had one wonderful day. Maybe we shouldn't ask for more than one such day in a lifetime."[38] Others, however, return to the drug again and again. The ancient Chinese sage Chuang Tzu once dreamt that he was a butterfly. In the dream he thought he had always been a butterfly, hovering amid the flowers. Then he awoke and was surprised to find that he was Chuang Tzu. But he could not be sure if he were really Chuang Tzu and had only dreamt that he was a butterfly, or if he were really a butterfly and was dreaming that he was Chuang Tzu.[39] To the chronic LSD user the border between the drug world and the real world may become very blurred. Another problem is the spontaneous recurrence of the LSD state, which may occur in a completely involuntary fashion and at the most inopportune times.

Cohen has also noted one very alarming aspect of the use of LSD in psychotherapy: the phenomenon of 'therapist breakdown'. Cohen found that an "unusual" number of those dispensing LSD as part of their therapy had themselves come down with psychiatric disorders. A "substantial" minority suffered from pronounced megalomania, depressions and psychotic behavior. Some had committed suicide. Cohen attributes this phenomenon to three factors: LSD had attracted those with somewhat unbalanced minds; LSD applied to other people is a powerful instrument for building one's own megalomania; the therapists in question had used the drug far too much themselves.[40] It is easy to see how the profound effects of the drug could lead the dispenser to view himself as a God-like creature, holding the life and death of individuals in his hands. It is also easy to see how Timothy Leary may have come to view himself, considering the following he attracted. Personally, I cannot escape the feeling that there is something wrong with anyone who *continues* to use LSD on a regular basis. If LSD unlocks new areas of the mind, then one should be able to continue the exploration without chemical aids. If the drug is continuously needed, this may be a sign that it is not doing its job, and ought to be abandoned. Otherwise its use will simply become an escape, an artificial means of substitution for normal adaptive behavior, in other words a form of drug dependency. LSD is a singularly inappropriate drug to be used as a crutch.

But what of its value in psychotherapy? We have tried to touch upon its wider philosophical values, and dangers, but the question remains concerning its specific efficacy as a tool of the medical profession. I am afraid that this question must go unanswered. Research projects are still underway and the results of the work already done are inconclusive. For example, LSD was used for years in Saskatchewan in the treatment of alcoholism. Results seemed to be encouraging. More long-range study is much less encouraging, however.[41] When and how LSD should be used is up to the specialists concerned. Unfortunately the popular hysteria and the legislative response have made the professional use of the drug not only much more difficult legally but also rather impolitic.

We have purposely left to the end the most serious criticism made against LSD, that its use causes damage to human chromosomes and may induce genetic defects in offspring. If this charge is true then it would seem that LSD could be as dangerous as thalidomide. But while the media have reported the dark side they have not reported as widely the contrary point of view. In fact the matter of chromosome damage is one of raging controversy among researchers.

One of the leading advocates of the view that LSD is genetically damaging is Dr. Maimon Cohen of Buffalo, New York. Dr. Cohen believes that he has found definite evidence of extensive damage to the chromosomes of human leukocytes (white blood cells), as well as to the leukocytes of babies whose mothers used LSD when pregnant. Dr. Cohen suggests that the production of congenital defects in offspring is entirely possible.[42] A group of pediatricians at the University of Iowa believe that they have encountered a well-documented case of an LSD-induced birth abnormality (a severely deformed right leg), and other research is presently being conducted into this possibility.[43] Further research with mice has also supported the hypothesis of chromosomal damage.[44]

The findings of some other researchers have been in direct conflict with the work already cited. One study of San Francisco hippie LSD users failed to confirm the Cohen findings.[45] A more recent study has also failed to demonstrate significant chromosomal damage among human subjects,[46] and some of the animal studies have also been challenged on the same basis.[47] Among the many problems involved would seem to be the question of whether the effect of LSD ingestion on isolated cells has any lasting effect. For example there is apparently some evidence that large amounts of aspirin or caffeine cause chromosomal damage. Does this mean that coffee-drinkers and aspirin users run the risk of extensive harm, or are the immediate effects merely transitory? Moreover it is not clear what precise meaning chromosomal breaks have for the organism. They are associated with leukemia, but whether as a cause or a by-product is a matter of some speculation. Nor does it seem at the moment that a causal link has been drawn between chromosome breakage and genetic defects in offspring.

I am not competent to carry this discussion any further. Suffice to say that any problem as subject to fierce debate among specialists as this one, is far from being resolved. At least a reasonable doubt has been created concerning the physical safety of LSD use. When such a doubt exists one might assume that the survival instinct of human beings would militate against the further use of such a possibly dangerous substance. Because the research emphasizing the genetic dangers of LSD has generally been carried out on a more intelligent and rational plane than much of the other anti-LSD work, it has consequently been given more weight by the users. In fact there is good evidence that beginning in 1968 the use of LSD began to decline, particularly among college students, although the hard-core hippies no doubt continue to be chronic users. It is my impression that the same thing has happened in Canada. It is interesting that the utter disdain with which anti-marijuana information is treated, contrasts sharply with the response to new information on LSD. This suggests that rationally-grounded educational programs may prove to be more useful than many government officials seem to expect. And certainly more effective than the kind of thing that happened in Pennsylvania, where a state official falsely reported that six college students had been permanently blinded by staring at the sun after taking LSD, and later had to resign after admitting publicly that the story was a complete hoax.[49]

We have now discussed at some length the question of what LSD is, how it works, and what it does. The subject is admittedly elusive and perplexing but it is difficult to see how it could be otherwise. We can now close out this discussion by turning to the legislative response to widespread LSD use in Canada.

In 1962, long before public concern was generally aroused, a new schedule was added to the Federal *Food and Drugs Act* listing two drugs, thalidomide and LSD. By amendment it was prescribed that "no person shall sell any drug" described in the new schedule.[50] Under the Act anyone violating any of its provisions is subject on summary conviction for a first offence to a $500 fine or three months imprisonment, or both, and for a subsequent offence, to $1000 or six months or both. On indictment, a defendant is subject to a $5000 fine or three years, or both. The Crown has the option of proceeding by either method.[51] While the RCMP have complained on many occasions that the LSD provision applies only to sales, and not to possession, the Act clearly defines "sell" as including "sell, offer for sale, expose for sale, *have in possession for sale*, and distribute".[52] (My italics.)

In 1967, the year that the LSD scare peaked, the legislatures of Alberta and British Columbia decided that the Federal law was insufficient and rushed to fill the breach. In Alberta, the *Public Health Act* was amended to make illegal the manufacture, distribution, possession, or the administration either to oneself or to others of an "hallucinogenic drug" (LSD or any other such substance as designated by the government). Violations could lead to fines and up to a year in prison.[53] By making the administration of a proscribed substance to oneself a criminal offence, Alberta thus went much further than most drug laws go even in the United States. At the same time the British Columbia legislature was so concerned about the problem that it actually passed *two* laws on the same subject in the same session of the legislature. *The Proscribed Substances Act* made it an offence to have LSD or marijuana in one's possession, subject to a $2000 fine or six months in prison, or both.[54] By the *Health Act Amendment Act*, unauthorized possession of LSD was to be penalized on the same basis as the Act previously referred to. But here it was also made an offence, subject to a $100 fine and six months in prison, or both, for "any person knowing of the presence of . . . LSD, in any premises or in the possession of any person" not to report such facts to the police.[55] The latter provision is, to put in mildly, somewhat unpalatable from a civil liberties standpoint.

The overlapping of jurisdictions inherent in legislating in areas already occupied by the Federal government came under attack in the courts. In Alberta an appeal against a conviction under the new *Public Health Act* amendment on the ground that the amendment was criminal law and therefore *ultra vires* of the province was rejected by the Alberta Supreme Court as well as by the appellate division.[56] In a similar case in British Columbia, an appeal was rejected in the Supreme Court chambers, with the Alberta decision as a guideline.[57] However, in October, 1968 the British Columbia Court of Appeal reversed this decision and granted the appeal, stating that the section in the *Health Act Amendment Act* making the possession of LSD an offence was clearly a provincial invasion of the criminal law field, and was thus *ultra vires* of the British Columbia legislature.[58]

The year 1967 also saw considerable agitation in Ottawa concerning LSD. In the Senate a bill was introduced that would make simple possession of LSD an offence as well as selling, and that would back the law with the same special police powers and burden of proof clauses, which we have earlier described as objectionable with regard to opiates and marijuana. Fulminating about the horrors of drugs and hippies proved to be as satisfying to the honorable Senators as attacking obscenity on the CBC, and once unleashed they proved to be more vigorous than their generally advanced age might indicate. Some points made by the Senators seem somewhat embarrassing in cold print. For example one speaker noted that "experiences of a religious mystical quality and a sense of communion with God also occur – as under the 'Arch Priest' Timothy Leary, the psychedelic exponent of the North American continent. He should be locked up!"[59] thus for the first and probably the last time lining up the Senate against God.

For reasons best known to the Senators, the bill was referred to the Banking and Commerce Committee, and it was here that things really got out of hand. Senator Molson of all persons – one might assume that the President of one of Canada's largest breweries would exhibit a certain diffidence in such matters – introduced an amendment, later passed by the Senate, which would make it a criminal offence subject to up to ten years imprisonment to "promote the use of or trafficking in a restricted drug". "Promotion" was to be defined by the Governor-in-Council.[60] Since the Senators had been waxing indignant about *Life* magazine, the CBC, and the *Perception '67* forum at the University of Toronto, the intent of this amendment was all too clear: the abolition of freedom of speech and of the press with regard to drug questions. And indeed one Senator went so far as to tell a television interviewer that promotion would mean "any favorable mention" about LSD, even by "word of mouth". Such an astonishing assault on the most basic liberties of Canadians drew a stern editorial rebuke from the Toronto *Globe and Mail*, which characterized the amendment as an attempt to "write into law one of the severest restrictions on freedom of expression and freedom of the press that has ever been contemplated in this country."[61] The Senators seemed quite unabashed by the criticism but when it became clear that the House of Commons was unlikely to pass such legislation the "promotion" clause was dropped at a later session.

By Order-in-Council in September 1968, the government added three new hallucinogenic drugs to the thalidomide-LSD schedule of the *Food and Drugs Act* (STP, DMT, and DET)[62] and two months later introduced Senate Bill S-15 for first reading in the House of Commons.[63] This legislation, which received royal assent in June of 1969, includes virtually the whole of the original 1967 Senate bill amending the *Food and Drugs Act*, with the exception of the "promotion" clause. STP, DMT, and DET were added to LSD on the schedule of 'restricted' drugs. Anyone guilty of possessing a restricted drug is subject, upon summary conviction for a first offence, to a fine of $1,000 or six months imprisonment, or both. A subsequent offence may be punished by a fine of $2,000 or one year in prison, or both. If the Crown chooses to proceed by indictment, the offender is subject to a fine of $5,000 or three years imprisonment, or both. Anyone found guilty of trafficking in a restricted drug – or of being in possession of such a drug for the purpose of trafficking – is liable, upon summary conviction, to eighteen months imprisonment or, upon conviction on indictment to ten years imprisonment.[64]

The problems raised by this type of legislation are numerous. The practical problems of enforcement are staggering since LSD, unlike marijuana, is colorless, odorless, tasteless, and potent in tiny amounts. It can be manufactured inside the country. Dr. Humphry Osmond of Princeton University, who along with Dr. Hoffer of Saskatchewan was one of the pioneers in LSD research, has suggested that there are no more than a half dozen persons in Canada qualified to certify that a substance is LSD, and cites a case in England where two defendants were acquitted of a charge of possessing LSD when a Nobel Prize-winning chemist and Dr. Albert Hofmann, the discoverer of LSD, were unable to agree on a technical definition of what LSD is. Another prominent American researcher in the field warned a meeting of the Ontario Medical and Ontario Psychiatric associations that United States laws had virtually halted private medical research, including his own, but that "the laws haven't stopped the people they most intended to combat – those who use LSD as a signal for rebellion against authority." He further suggested that Canada might learn from the United States situation.[65]

It is not necessary to rehearse once again all the arguments raised against the legal treatment of marijuana users except to suggest that all such arguments apply equally to LSD. In fact the 'lottery' aspect of law enforcement is worsened in the case of LSD, because of the detection problems. It is most depressing to see the special police powers and the burden of proof procedures being applied to yet another category of drugs. The progress of anti-drug laws begins to seem like a steady rout of a host of personal rights and liberties.

On the other hand, we have already suggested that LSD *is* dangerous and we cannot in all conscience conclude that LSD or other powerful hallucinogenics should be allowed free distribution. There are at least three separate grounds for controlling such drugs: the mental dangers to individuals, the physical dangers to individuals, and the social dangers. It seems that many people with deep psychological disorders turn to LSD as a 'solution' to their problems, but these are precisely the people least able to handle the experience. Yet it is difficult to see how tough laws will in themselves discourage such use, since such persons are not likely to act rationally toward either drugs or laws. Moreover, these people are the ones who most need medical help, not punishment. As for the question of physical damage, the evidence concerning chromosomal breakages is not yet solid enough to build a statute upon. However, if irrefutable proof of genetic damage is forthcoming, the libertarian defence of drug use – that it does not harm anyone else – largely collapses. The State has a clear duty to intervene to protect the rights of future children who may be born with congenital defects.

The social dangers fall into two categories. First of all, there are the specific dangers to other individuals. A person driving a car while undergoing an LSD experience is even more dangerous than a driver smoking marijuana. Some persons have turned violent and even homicidal while under the influence of LSD. A man in New York who stabbed his mother to death was acquitted by reason of temporary insanity induced by LSD. It is my strongly-held belief that this is a disastrous judicial doctrine, for it not only dispenses with the question of the individual's moral responsibility in voluntarily consuming a drug that he knows will induce unpredictable behavior, but it also encourages a careless attitude toward the consequences of drug use. It is thus to be hoped that a recent decision in the district court of Sudbury, Ontario will constitute an important precedent for all such cases. In *Regina v. MacIsaac*, the defendant was charged with four counts of robbery, attempted robbery, breaking and entering. His defence was that he was at all times under the influence of LSD and was therefore not responsible for his actions. The judge concluded that the accused was not in fact under the influence of LSD; he was also at pains to point out that

> Having regard to the widespread publicity given to LSD and the notoriety of its effects and having regard to the age and background of the accused including the prior use of marijuana, the only reasonable conclusion is that before taking the LSD he not only knew of its effects but intended and desired to attain the state produced by the drug.
>
> In view of this finding I come to the conclusion that, in line with the decisions above mentioned, the voluntary consumption of LSD like the voluntary consumption of alcohol, is not a defence to any of the charges in this indictment.[66]

We will return to this question in the final chapter.

Finally, there is a second face to the problem of social dangers that is by no means so clear-cut. It is obvious from reading the debates in Parliament and in the provincial legislatures that to many lawmakers, the hallucinogenic drugs pose a subversive threat to the fabric of our civilization. No doubt a certain threat does exist and while I personally do not share the fear of the guardians of established order, I can nevertheless understand their motives. But the final truth in this regard is that the problem transcends the ability of legislatures to control it through specific outlawing of specific drugs. For as Dr. Abram Hoffer has suggested, it is the *experience*, not the drug, that people seek. As we shall see in the next chapter there already exists a vast proliferation of naturally-occurring hallucinogenic substances some of which would be very difficult to outlaw. Moreover, as we pointed out earlier, the methods used by religious mystics, such as breathing deeply to concentrate carbon dioxide in the brain, have nothing to do with drugs. The two personal experiences I recounted were brought about by a hospital anaesthetic and unusual climatic conditions. As Dr. Hoffer points out, the LSD-type experience can be achieved by

hypnosis, sensory deprivation, sleeplessness, environmental manipulations using vivid visual and auditory stimuli plus rhythm in which the psychedelic seeker participates actively. One can also use starvation in a cave, physical exhaustion, prolonged contemplation. It is also likely that in the near future newer non-drug methods will be developed. . . . It will be just as difficult to control these experiences as it is to control a man from thinking.[67]

Ban deep breathing? Ban sleeplessness? Ban music? Ban contemplation? Ban religion? Will this be the legislative agenda for the 1970s? LSD and the other powerful hallucinogenics carry with them their own specific dangers and some form of control must be exercised. But let no-one be deluded that such controls will eliminate the type of experience induced by the drugs. And why ultimately should we try to eliminate such experience? Are we afraid that the discovery of other levels of consciousness will betray the inadequacies of the established view of life? And is that a worthy motive?

Footnotes

[1]One such attempt is in William Marshall and Gilbert W. Taylor, *The Art of Ecstasy: an Investigation of the Psychedelic Revolution* (Toronto, Burns and MacEachern, 1967), based on the *Perception '67* symposium at the University of Toronto.

[2]Humphry Osmond, "A Review of the Clinical Effects of Psychotomimetic Agents," in David Solomon, ed., *LSD: The Consciousness-Expanding Drug* (New York, G. P. Putnam's Sons, 1964), pp. 128-51.

[3]This account is drawn mainly from R. E. L. Masters and Jean Houston, *The Varieties of Psychedelic Experience* (New York, Delta Books, 1967), pp. 49-50.

[4]Nicholas J. Giarman, "The Pharmacology of LSD," in Richard C. DeBold and Russell C. Leaf, eds., *LSD, Man, and Society* (Middletown, Connecticut, Wesleyan University Press, 1967), pp. 143-44.

[5]Sidney Cohen, *The Beyond Within: The LSD Story,* 2nd ed. (New York, Atheneum, 1967), pp. 36-37.

[6]An imaginative statement and elaboration of this concept may be found in Kenneth Boulding, *The Image: Knowledge in Life and Society* (Ann Arbor, Michigan, University of Michigan Press, 1961).

[7]J. Bronowski, "The Machinery of Nature," *Encounter,* vol. XXV, no. 5 (November, 1965), p. 48.

[8]A lucid explanation of the mechanism of the synapse can be found in E. G. Gray, "The Synapse," *Science Journal,* vol. 3, no. 5 (May, 1967), pp. 66-72.

[9]Giarman, *op. cit.,* p. 147.

[10]George K. Aghajanian, Warren E. Foote, Michael H. Sheard, "Lysergic Acid Diethylamide: Sensitive Neuronal Units in the Midbrain Raphe," *Science,* vol. 161 (August 16, 1968), pp. 706-8.

[11]Dominick P. Purpura, "Neurophysiological actions of LSD," in DeBold and Leaf, *op. cit.,* p. 182.

[12]See footnote (8) above.

[13]Allen Ginsberg, "Christmas on Earth: Remarks on Leary's Politics of Ecstasy," *The Village Voice* (December 12, 1968), p. 6.

[14]Cohen, *op. cit.,* pp. 200-201.

[15]K. H. Blacker, R. Jones, A. Stone, and D. Pfefferbaum, "Chronic Users of LSD: The 'Acidheads'," *American Journal of Psychiatry,* vol. 125, no. 3 (September, 1968), pp. 341-51.

[16]Charles Clay Dahlberg, "LSD Psychotherapy," *The Village Voice* (January 9, 1969), p. 22.

[17]C. A. Doxiadis, "Man's Movement and his City," *Science,* vol. 162 (October 18, 1968), p. 331.

[18]Albert Einstein, *Relativity: The Special and the General Theory,* 15th ed. (London, Methuen and Co., 1960), p. 141.

[19]Masters and Houston, *op. cit.,* p. 127.

[20]William Burroughs, "Academy 23: a Deconditioning," *The Village Voice* (July 6, 1967), p. 21.

[21]Alan W. Watts, *The Joyous Cosmology: Adventures in the Chemistry of Consciousness* (New York, Random House, 1962). See also "The New Alchemy" in Watts, *This is It, and Other Essays* (New York, Collier Books, 1967), pp. 125-53.

[22]Aldous Huxley, *The Doors of Perception* and *Heaven and Hell* (Harmondsworth, Middlesex, Penguin Books, 1959).

[23]William James, *The Varieties of Religious Experience: a Study in Human Nature* (New York, New American Library, 1958). First published in 1902.

[24]Timothy Leary, Ralph Metzner, Richard Alpert, *The Psychedelic Experience: a manual based on the Tibetan Book of the Dead.* (New Hyde Park, New York, University Books, 1964). W. Y. Evans-Wentz, ed., *The Tibetan Book of the Dead* (New York, Oxford University Press, 1960). First published, 1927.

[25]R. M. Bucke, *Cosmic Consciousness: a Study in the Evolution of the Human Mind,* quoted in James, *op. cit.,* pp. 306-7.

[26]*Ibid.,* p. 298.

[27]Huxley, *Doors of Perception,* op. cit., p. 24.

[28]Huxley, *Heaven and Hell,* op. cit., pp. 121-22.

[29]Simone de Beauvoir, *La force de l'âge* (Paris, Librairie Gallimard, 1960), pp. 216-18.

[30]William Braden, *The Private Sea: LSD and The Search for God* (New York, Bantam Books, 1968), p. 167.

[31]M. A. Sèchehaye, *Autobiography of a Schizophrenic Girl* (New York, Grune and Stratton, 1951). The original French phrase was 'le pays d'éclairement'.

[32]Thomas S. Szasz, *The Myth of Mental Illness* (New York, Hoeber-Harper, 1961).

[33]Michel Foucault, *Histoire de la folie à l'âge classique* (Paris, Librairie Plon, 1961). Freud once told Jung that his sexual theory must be made into a

"dogma, an unshakable bulwark" against the "black tide of mud, of occultism". C. G. Jung, *Memories, Dreams, Reflections* (New York, Pantheon Books, 1961), p. 150. Freud was himself engaged in excavating the irrational elements of the mind but he was also attempting to control these elements by placing them within a rigid scientific framework. The paradox is acute, and very suggestive of what Foucault means by the relationship of the rational to the non-rational.

[34]R. D. Laing, *The Politics of Experience* and *The Bird of Paradise* (Harmondsworth, Middlesex, Penguin Books, 1967), p. 105.

[35]See Herbert Marcuse, *An Essay on Liberation* (Boston, Beacon Press, 1969), pp. 36-37 and 83-84.

[36]N. Cohn, *The Pursuit of the Millennium* (London, Secker and Warburg, 1961), pp. 314-18.

[37]*Ibid.*, pp. 273-74.

[38]Cohen, *op. cit.*, p. 140.

[39]Arthur Waley, *Three Ways of Thought in Ancient China* (Garden City, New York, Doubleday and Company, 1956), p. 32.

[40]Cohen, *op. cit.*, pp. 217-19.

[41]See, for example, Reginald C. Smart *et al.*, *Lysergic Acid Diethylamide (LSD) in the Treatment of Alcoholism* (Toronto, University of Toronto Press, 1967).

[42]M. M. Cohen, "LSD and Chromosomes," *Science Journal*, vol. 4, no. 9 (September, 1968), pp. 76-79.

[43]"Doctors blame LSD for baby's defects," *The Globe and Mail* (November 24, 1967).

[44]See, for example, N. E. Skakkbaek, J. Philip, O. J. Rafaelsen, "LSD in Mice: Abnormalities in Meiotic Chromosomes," *Science*, vol. 160, (1968), pp. 1246-48.

[45]W. D. Loughman *et al.*, "Leukocytes of humans exposed to lysergic acid diethylamide: lack of chromosomal damage," *Science*, vol. 158 (1967), p. 308.

[46]Robert S. Sparkes *et al.*, "Chromosomal Effect in vivo of exposure to lysergic acid diethylamide," *Science*, vol. 160 (1968), pp. 1343-45. But see also the criticisms of this study as well as the authors' reply in *Science*, vol. 162 (1968), pp. 1508-9.

[47]Dale Grace *et al.*, "Drosophila melanogaster treated with LSD: absence of mutation and chromosome breakage," *Science*, vol. 161 (1968), pp. 694-96.

[48]Douglas Robinson, "U.S. Drug Authorities say LSD levelling off," *The Globe and Mail* (March 5, 1968).

[49]"Story of college students blinded by sun a hoax, governor says," *The Globe and Mail* (January 14, 1968). "No prosecution in LSD hoax, state decides," *ibid.* (January 31, 1968).

[50]11 Eliz. II (1962-63), c. 15, s. 14(A).

[51]1-2 Eliz. II (1952-53), c. 38, s. 25.

[52]*Ibid.*, c. 38, s. 2(M).

[53]Statutes of Alberta, 16 Eliz. II (1967), c. 63.

[54]RSBC, 15-16 Eliz. II (1967), c. 37.

[55]RSBC, 15-16 Eliz. II (1967), c. 21.

[56]*R. v. Snyder and Fletcher* (1967) 61 WWR, 112. Confirmed at 61 WWR, 576.

[57]*R. v. Simpson et al*, (1968) 63 WWR, 606.

[58]*Simpson et al v. R.*, (1969) 66 WWR, 621.

[59]Senate of Canada, *Debates* (April 19, 1967), p. 1797.

[60]Minutes of the Proceedings of the Senate of Canada, (April 26, 1967), p. 1373.

[61]"Some senatorial fantasies," *The Globe and Mail* (May 1, 1967), p. 6.

[62]P.C. 1968-1736 (September 25, 1968).

[63]House of Commons, *Debates* (November 21, 1968), p. 3004.

[64]17-18 Eliz. II (1969) c. 41, ss. 39-45.

[65]"LSD laws in U.S. described as hindrance," *The Globe and Mail* (May 12, 1967). The speaker was Dr. Harold Abramson of New York.

[66]*R. v. MacIsaac*, Sudbury District Court (November 8, 1968). Reported in *The Criminal Law Quarterly*, vol. 11, no. 2 (February, 1969), pp. 234-40.

[67]Abram Hoffer, "Why suppression of LSD won't curb psychedelia," *The Globe and Mail* (July 21, 1967), p. 7. This article originally appeared as "Psychedelic experiences and the Law" in *Chitty's Law Journal*, vol. 15, no. 6 (June 1967), pp. 182-88. See also the same author's "Confrontation between the psychedelic experience and society," *Canadian Dimension*, vol. 4, no. 5 (Summer, 1967), pp. 5-7. Robert de Ropp has elaborated an entire book around the non-drug exploration of the self: de Ropp, *The Master Game: Pathways to Higher Consciousness Beyond the Drug Experience* (New York, Delta Books, 1969).

The World's Biggest Drugstore

7

Mother Nature is the world's worst dope pusher. From the lonely steppes of Siberia to the humid jungles of Central America, from the sun-burnt deserts of the American southwest to the gardens of little old ladies in Toronto, she has thoughtfully placed in our path a myriad of plants that when ingested, can cause stimulation, depression, euphoria, insanity, ecstasy, idiocy, and addiction. It is difficult enough to stop the manufacture of synthetic drugs, but to try to ban naturally occurring plants is legislative bravado on a truly awesome scale. And even with the synthetics, the prohibitionist legislator faces a formidable task of banning any number of new substances as soon as they appear.

We might begin with the hallucinogenics, although in reality this category is an elastic one; since so many young drug users actively seek out hallucinatory experiences, it is not surprising that a wide variety of substances have been found to induce such effects. By the same token, the same substances have induced other effects in those who are not looking for hallucinations in the first place. Amphetamines have been described as hallucinogenic. Some teen-agers have even reported hallucinating after ingesting tranquillizers and sleeping pills. In advanced stages of alcoholism, the condition known as *delirium tremens* often occurs: the famous 'pink elephants' are one product of this state of mind; other much less benign hallucinations may take shape. But purely pharmacological considerations to the side, it is evident that a number of substances are being used mainly for hallucinogenic *purposes*, and these we can examine.

The biggest single problem in discussing the commonly-used hallucinogenics is that of contamination. Since the distribution of these drugs is entirely a black market affair there is no quality control, and no supervisory agency to inspect the goods and certify their contents. The cannabis situation is very bad in this regard, but the 'acid' situation is much worse. Since synthetic hallucinogenics come in such tiny doses, the ordinary user has no way of knowing what he has bought until he tries it – and then, in all too many cases, it may be too late. A few years ago it was widely reported that any high-school student with a chemistry set could synthesize his own LSD. In fact it appears to be much more complicated than that, but this does not prevent shoddy and dangerous material from being produced and sold as LSD.

Recently a confidential analysis prepared by the Addiction Research Foundation of Ontario based on collected street samples found that there are four types of LSD currently being sold, only one of which is free of impurities. Incomplete synthesis can apparently lead to a concentration of toxic substances. The Foundation's confidential report found its way into the hands of the Toronto drug subculture where, amusingly enough, it served as a kind of Consumers' Report for acid-heads.[1] For anyone genuinely concerned about the safety of young drug users this development should be taken, not as a cause for bureaucratic chagrin, but as an example of what a government can really do to 'help' the user.

Another danger lurking in black market LSD is the inclusion of strychnine, which, in small doses, is capable of causing stimulation, but is also a deadly poison. *Ergot*, the grain fungus in which natural lysergic acid is found, is the cause of a terrible disease known as St. Anthony's Fire, in which the extremities of the body turn a gangrenous black and fall off. If LSD is properly synthesized and properly stored the dangers of poisoning should be almost nonexistent. But it is quite probable that a good proportion of the well-publicized 'bad trips', and much of the permanent mental damage that has followed LSD use, has been a result not of LSD itself but of the impurities it contains. In street jargon, when someone buys a drug that purports to be something it is not, the buyer has been 'burned'. There have been a lot of people burned, both figuratively and literally. The dictionary defines *acid* as a *sour substance*: the name thus befits a lot of the products sold on the streets today. Just as there are 'heroin-addicts' who are not really addicted to heroin but to the harmless milk-sugar sold as heroin, so there may be 'acid-heads' who have never really taken genuine LSD. Here is something that the Department of Consumer Affairs could look into!

There are a number of chemical variants of LSD. Mescalin is an active agent in the peyote cactus, and psilocybin is derived from a Mexican mushroom; we will discuss these later, but they do not seem to be used illicitly in Canada to any extent. More important are entirely synthetic creations, such as DET (N, N-Diethyltryptamine) and DMT (N, N-Dimethyltryptamine). DMT is a somewhat milder form of LSD, the effects only lasting for about a half hour. Most important of all is a drug commonly known as STP. These letters do not have any chemical meaning, but apparently are derived from 'Serenity', 'Tranquillity', and 'Peace' – although another story is that the name was adopted so that advantage could be taken of "STP" decals handed out as promotional material by a company marketing an automotive additive of that name. In any event something going under the label *STP* made its black market appearance in the late spring of 1967 and soon gained a reputation as being to regular LSD what the hydrogen bomb is to the atom bomb. It is quite probable that more than one substance has been sold as STP, but it now seems that the basic form is a compound known as 4-Methyl-2, 5-dimethoxyamphetamine or DOM. This is a formula, related to both mescaline and amphetamine, that was developed by Dow Chemical Co. for possible use in the treatment of mental illness. In very small doses the drug is apparently not very harmful, and may even have a certain clinical usefulness,[2] but in the large dosages in which illicit users confront it, STP is a very dangerous drug indeed. Although closely guarded by the company, the formula somehow slipped out[3] and became a novelty in North American drug subcultures for a time. Its use seems to have tapered off considerably, however, as its ill effects became known. The mixture of mescalin and amphetamine is a strange brew. The effects may last up to four or five days, and the amphetamine content causes prolonged sleeplessness throughout the period. Unlike LSD, there have been reports that STP ingestion has caused fatal physiological complications. Moreover, some of the violent and paranoiac symptoms of prolonged amphetamine use have been reported in connection with STP. Happily the drug users themselves seem to be aware of this. STP, DMT, and DET are included along with LSD in the new category of 'restricted drugs' recently added to the *Food and Drugs Act*.

Two varieties of Morning Glory – appropriately called *Pearly Gates* and *Heavenly Blue* – produce seeds that contain alkaloids of lysergic acid.[4] Soon after this fact became known, seed suppliers reported a hitherto unnoticed interest in gardening by long-haired youth. A young American student chewed 300 such seeds and went into a prolonged psychotic state, which ended weeks later when he drove his car down a hill at 100 m.p.h. and crashed into a house, killing himself.[5] Often, however, the effects are so mild that the hopeful users have been disappointed – probably because they failed to chew the seeds properly. In addition, agricultural authorities have begun spraying the seeds with pesticides and nausea-producing chemicals to discourage their use,[6] although any really dedicated experimenter could presumably grow his own seeds. The chewing of Morning Glory seeds as part of religious rituals is a very old practice in Mexico. Hermández, a royal physician in sixteenth-century Spain, witnessed Aztec priests eating such seeds when they wished to commune with their gods: "a thousand visions and satanic hallucinations appeared to them".[7] It is difficult to imagine any possible way that governments could altogether stop this practice. One imagines ordinary gardeners rising up in righteous indignation against any such attempt, and bizarre scenes of narcotics agents ripping out the gardens of protesting old ladies!

Another hallucinogenic that it is difficult to imagine being banned is one found in almost every kitchen and spice-rack – nutmeg. This spice, along with a similar spice called *mace*, if taken in sufficient quantity can bring about effects that can, on occasion, rival those of LSD, although the results are quite variable, depending on the type of nutmeg and quantity used. There are usually unpleasant side effects, such as headache, dizziness, and nausea.[8] There are reports that a synthesis of nutmeg, called MDA, has gone into illicit circulation, but at the moment little is known about this substance or its effects. In any event, there is nothing to prevent anyone, of any age, buying as much nutmeg as they want at the local supermarket. What is more, the use of nutmeg as a spice in cooking is so well established that its use for other purposes will simply have to be lived with.

Mescalin, which is derived from peyote, is close to LSD. The buttons of the peyote cactus will have the same effects as mescalin if swallowed. The peyote cactus grows wild in central and northern Mexico, but its use as a religious sacrament by North American Indians extends up to Saskatchewan. It seems to have been of great value to the Indians as part of an effort at cultural regroupment after the first shattering impact of the white man, but it should be noted –

especially by hippies – that its use by the Indians is rigidly controlled within a set of well-defined rituals, and has nothing hedonistic about it.[9] One problem that adventurous white experimenters have run into is that peyote has a terrible taste. It takes a good deal of single-minded dedication to swallow and keep down the tough and nauseating buttons. William James was long ago intrigued by accounts he had heard of peyote experiences. "The great psychologist consumed one button, was 'violently sick for twenty-four hours', emerged with an horrendous hangover and advised brother Henry that 'I will take the visions on trust'."[10]

Another potent natural hallucinogenic is the so-called 'magic mushroom'. When Alice was journeying through Wonderland she came upon a caterpillar sitting atop a mushroom and smoking a hookah. The caterpillar informed her that if she ate one side of the mushroom it would make her tall, and if she ate the other side it would make her small. Many people besides Alice have had strange experiences with mushrooms. There are apparently a number that grow in Mexico that have hallucinogenic properties. Psilocybin, a drug whose effects are quite similar to LSD, although milder, is derived from a Mexican mushroom. The *fly agaric*, so called because of its use to poison flies, is used by native peoples in Siberia for religious intoxication. Since the intoxicating agents pass unaltered through the body in the urine, the unusual practice of drinking each other's urine makes possible an indefinite prolongation of the desired state, when it is used in groups.[11]

In South America a vine called *Banisteria Caapi* is an hallucinogenic whose potency, by all reports, is similar to that of LSD. *Yage*, as the Indians call it, has one very peculiar property: the color blue seems to be almost always associated with its hallucinatory effects.

One of the strangest of these natural drugs is found in the *Solanaceae* family of plants. Datura, belladonna, mandragora, mandrake, henbane, Jimson weed, Devil weed, deadly nightshade, stramonium – these are some of the names and forms of this group of plants whose properties seem to have frightened and fascinated human beings in many countries and many ages. It was apparently associated with the Bacchanalian orgies of ancient Greece and with the witch cult in the Middle Ages. Some 300 years ago a British army company camped near Jamestown, Virginia, and prepared a stew with some local greens, among which was the Jimson (Jamestown) weed. The results were an eleven day period of innocent madness. When rubbed on the body as a paste, it induces visions of flying – in various cultures the same imagery occurs, interestingly enough. In Asia, Africa and the Americas it has been used as an intoxicant by native peoples. Unfortunately, as its various names indicate, datura has a high potential for toxicity. Worse, it has the reputation of being a capricious and unpredictable drug, and for this reason is widely feared.[12]

Recently six young people in Toronto were admitted to hospital in a raving, screaming state of temporary insanity. The cause apparently was stramonium, obtained from drugstores. A fourteen-year-old boy died in Guelph after suffering convulsions; it was thought that stramonium was to blame.[13] Asthmador, a non-prescription remedy for asthma symptoms, contains stramonium and other belladonna alkaloids, and is easily available.[14] But once again, while tightening of pharmaceutical procedures could cut down on the easy availability of the drug, *Solanaceae* plants grow all over the world.

As Aldous Huxley has remarked, there seem to be no plants with intoxicating properties that have not been known since time immemorial.[15] While cannabis and narcotic type plants have often been used to excess, and purely for purposes of 'drowning sorrows', it is an interesting and significant fact that among the so-called 'primitive' people, the more strictly hallucinogenic plants have usually been treated with a great deal of respect, and their use tends to be bound up with religious ritual. Frivolous, thrill-seeking use of such drugs seems to be much more of a contemporary Western problem. Carlos Castenada, a young anthropology student at Berkeley, has written a compelling account of his experiences as the pupil of Don Juan, an old Indian *brujo*, or teacher, who with the use of peyote, datura, and psilocybin, attempted to bring him into the state of 'non-ordinary reality', a higher plane of consciousness. The use of each of these drugs was accompanied by the most elaborate forms of ritual in their gathering, preparation, and use.[16] It may well be that precisely this lack of a structured, ritualistic setting has caused so much of the confusion and trouble concerning psychedelic drugs in contemporary society. In most non-Western cultures, the ecstatic, shamanistic, non-rational qualities of the human mind have a traditional and accepted place. The use of hallucinogenic drugs 'fits' culturally into this context; in the West, however, their use becomes perforce a rebellion against the cultural domination of rationalism, science, and technology. Too often this rebellion has been a simple-minded search for mere novelty, and its results chaotic and meaningless.

Despite this unfortunate fact, it is not likely that the use of hallucinogens is merely a passing fad. I think rather that the current fashion has touched a very raw nerve in the Western world outlook, one that will continue to be agitated by young people who dimly recognize a basic emotional deficiency in the world around them. The sensual, orgiastic rhythms of rock music are one answer to this need; ecstatic drug experiences are another. The truly sane answer to this fact may well be to accommodate our civilization to the impulse, rather than to try to stamp out the impulse for the sake of preserving the civilization unchanged. But we can be sure that such an accommodation will only come after a great struggle; drug users are sure to be among the chief victims of this struggle, victims not only of laws and repression, but of their own silly excesses as well.

Many of the needs that such drugs appear to fulfill can be met in other ways, but our civilization rarely approves of these other means any more than it does of drug taking. The old Roman *Saturnalia* was a long festival of freedom in which duties were cast aside and music, merry-making, and laughter prevailed. The idea of the *Mardi Gras* remains today, although in places of Latin origin, such as Rio de Janeiro and New Orleans. Quebec has its *carnival*, but the best we dour English Canadians can offer is the rather sad drunken chauvinism of Grey Cup weekend. A real carnival would be a harmless, colorful, orgiastic, ritual violation of all the prohibitions of society. As Paul and Percival Goodman have explained: "By day-to-day acquiescence and cooperation, people put on the habit of some society or other. . . . Meantime, submerged impulses of excess and destruction gather force and periodically explode in wild public holidays or gigantic wars (there is also occasional private collapse)." The answer, the Goodmans suggest, would be a "season of carnival, when the boundaries are overriden between zone and zone, and the social order is loosed to the equalities and inequalities of nature".[17] The celebrated May Revolution in France in 1968 was in many ways less of a revolution than just such a carnival, a 'festival of the oppressed' as some have called it. The fact that every teenage rock show threatens to turn into either an orgy or a riot is an illustration of the same phenomenon. Smoking pot and taking acid trips is another. One wonders how much of the ugliness and violence betrayed by both sides in demonstrations and riots is the result of the repressions of a society that never relaxes its strict supervision of all its citizens' activities. Alan Watts writes that:

No one is more dangerously insane than one who is sane all the time:
he is like a steel bridge without flexibility, and the order of his life is rigid
and brittle. The manners and mores of Western civilization force this
perpetual sanity upon us to an extreme degree, for there is no accepted
corner in our lives for the art of pure nonsense ...

If our sanity is to be strong and flexible, there must be occasional
periods for the expression of completely spontaneous movement – for
dancing, singing, howling, babbling, jumping, groaning, wailing – in short,
for following any motion to which the organism as a whole seems to be
inclined. It is by no means impossible to set up physical and moral
boundaries within which this freedom of action is expressible ...[18]

Until this concept is understood there is little point in trying to understand the motives of kids taking hallucinogens. Providing other channels for such impulses would probably diminish, rather than increase, drug use; but one cannot escape the feeling that it is the impulses, more than the drugs, that the guardians of law and order and public decency most fear.

So much for the hallucinogens. Some might dismiss the last few paragraphs as being irrelevant. I think not. The hallucinogens have always been bound up with the deeper religious and philosophical mysteries of human existence. To discuss them in complete isolation from such considerations would be as misleading as a discussion of sex without any mention of its profound relationship to the human psyche. But as we move on from the hallucinogens to other forms of youthful drug use we get into activities that are not only more crudely thrill-seeking in nature, but more self-destructive as well.

The amphetamine situation is today a very ugly scene, perhaps the worst in the entire spectrum of contemporary youthful drug abuse, worse in many ways than the world of the heroin addict. Sometimes used in conjunction with LSD – as a kind of *ad hoc* form of STP – amphetamines (*speed*) are increasingly used by themselves. Amphetamines are, as the name *speed* implies, stimulant drugs that cause bursts of energy. Sometimes used clinically to combat narcolepsy (a disease in which the subject is constantly falling asleep), to induce euphoria in extremely depressed persons, or to diminish appetite, amphetamines have long been familiar to students studying for final exams. In the form of Benzedrine (Bennies) and Dexedrine

(Dexies), amphetamines have became a familiar part of middle-class life, providing a lift when a lift is needed. Unfortunately they also have many ill effects, of which severe depressions after the stimulation wears off is the most immediately noticeable. For example, I have known fellow students at university who studied without sleep for several days on pep pills. In more than one instance the effects wore off while an examination was being written: the results were depression, malaise, and a catastrophic decline in the quality of their answers. Amphetamines rob the body's energy bank; but accounts must be paid eventually.

That amphetamine misuse could cause serious problems has been known for some time. A very serious problem arose in post-war Japan among adolescents, and in Britain their use by teen-agers for weekend stimulation has been a problem for a number of years. In North America isolated cases of amphetamine dependency and amphetamine psychosis have been coming to the attention of health authorities for a number of years, but such cases do not seem to be part of an organized subculture of amphetamine use. Dr. O. J. Kalant has prepared an extensive survey of existing medical knowledge concerning the effects of amphetamines for the Ontario Addiction Research Foundation. She summarizes the undesirable side of these drugs as follows:

1. Acute toxic states characterized by symptoms of overstimulation of the sympathetic and central nervous systems. The severity of the symptoms depends on the dose and on the susceptibility of the individual and can range from mild states of euphoria through acute psychotic reactions of a paranoid type to death ...

2. Various degrees of dependence ranging from mild habituation to strong compulsion to using the drugs chronically. The more severe cases of dependence show all the characteristics of true addiction.

3. The development of marked tolerance leading to the need for increased doses, with marked chronic undesirable side effects such as insomnia, anorexia, and abnormal behavior.

4. The development of transitory psychotic reactions clinically indistinguishable from paranoid schizophrenia. These toxic psychoses can occur both as a result of single doses of amphetamines and in chronic users of the drugs. In the latter the prognosis is bad in the sense that the risk of recurrence is directly related to the continued consumption of amphetamines.

5. Damage to society in the form of neglect of family and work, financial irresponsibility, crime, and other anti-social behavior.[19]

But the problems pointed up by excessive use of amphetamine pills or inhalers are only part of the trouble. In the past few years members of the drug subcultures have begun the practice of injecting methadrine directly into the veins. This greatly intensifies both the pleasurable feelings and the destructive effects. Immediately after injection, a 'flash', an overwhelming feeling of pleasure – somewhat like an orgasm spreading over the body – is experienced, followed by a long period of euphoric and compulsive activity. Coming down from this state is, however, a dreaded event and therefore methadrine is continuously injected to put off the inevitable moment of reckoning. Eventually, after perhaps a week at the utmost, the utterly exhausted user can go no further and sinks into a depressive condition of withdrawal. *Meth heads* or *speed freaks* present a number of problems in more acute form than those presented by the conventional amphetamine users. Needles used for injection are often dirty, and used communally, thus giving rise to outbreaks of infectious hepatitis in hippie communities. The tolerance mechanism means that increasing dosages are necessary. While a clinical dose may run between 5 to 30 milligrams a day, the meth head may shoot up to 300 milligrams every few hours for a number of days.[20] Since amphetamine depresses the appetite, the user may suffer severe loss of weight. Although there is much debate on this matter, methadrine injection would seem to lead to a physiological condition very much like addiction. Electroencephalographic readings of brain waves during sleep show a major disturbance after the withdrawal of the drug, which may last up to eight weeks.[21] Three doctors who studied methadrine use in California concluded that "the amphetamine users are impelled to return to use of their drug with a force comparable to that of heroin users."[22] The same study found an even more alarming effect: about one-third of the users they studied closely admitted that their memory and ability to concentrate had suffered permanent damage.

Speed freaks are unpopular people, particularly with those unfortunate enough to be friends or acquaintances. Hippie communities such as Yorkville and Haight-Ashbury are filled with wasted speed freaks, sick and paranoiac and avoided by all. Nobody is more worried by the speed plague than the hallucinogenic drug users and the genuine hippies, who see speed not only as a destructive addiction, but as a violation of the entire ethic built up around the use of cannabis and LSD as mind-expanding aids. Speed is, quite literally, mind-destroying rather than mind-expanding. And its chronic use brings out in extreme form the very personality characteristics that the use of pot and acid is supposed to counteract: ceaseless aggressive activity, egocentric intolerance of others, greediness, and violent paranoia. SPEED KILLS! warn posters and buttons put out not by the police or the government but by young drug users themselves, who have a first-hand knowledge of just how killing the drug can be.

In the summer of 1967 a sixty-six year old man was driving in Connecticut and noticed a parked car with a girl's head resting in the window. He stopped and asked her if she was all right, but a young man who emerged from beside the girl dragged the older man out of his car, threw him to the ground, beat him, and twisted off his left foot so that only a piece of flesh connected it to his leg. Attempts to re-attach the foot in hospital were unsuccessful. The assailant pleaded in court that he was under the influence of amphetamine and did not know what he was doing. He was given a sentence of from two to eight years in prison.[23] Of course the story about amphetamines may have been no more than a *post facto* excuse, but such a revolting act of violence has been matched by stories from hippie communities of sudden senseless assaults and murders committed by speed freaks. After recognizing how overdrawn such stories were when attributed to cannabis, one must be wary. But what is most chilling about speed is that nobody seems to have anything positive to say about the drug; the speed freaks themselves quickly become addicted and lose any free choice in the matter. A high-school dropout at first found life exciting when shooting meth. But when the inevitable 'bringdown' kept recurring and when his friends had all closed their doors to him because of his constant thefts, he locked himself in his room for days, bashing his head against the wall to fight the need for more. Eventually he went back to it: he knows what it does to him and does not attempt to justify its use. It is nothing more nor less than a compulsion. And the future of a speed freak is dim. Anybody who shoots 200 to 300 milligrams of methadrine every few hours for several days around the clock, quite probably has a low life expectancy. Some have suggested five years at the most. Unfortunately hard scientific data on meth freaks is difficult to come by. One hopes that much more will be done, for such data is certainly needed.

Strangely enough, parliament and the press, despite their (sometimes hysterical) concern over cannabis and LSD, have not been

overly exercised by the use of speed. Nor do the police seem as concerned about methadrine as they are about pot. Of course pot is a
more attractive target for law enforcement than speed – it is bulkier,
more distinctive in form and smell, and less easily disguised. Some
writers in the underground press have suggested – I hope they are
wrong – that the establishment is not so worried about speed because
the personality effects associated with its use are more in keeping
with North American values, than those associated with the more
passive and introspective users of cannabis and LSD. To rephrase the
point somewhat, it might be said that speed freaks may not be quite
as *visible* as the acid-heads, with their exotic costumes and bizarre
hair styles. Moreover the cannabis and LSD users tend to be much
more articulate about their drug habits; the real meth head does not
go about promoting his particular affliction. Finally, one rather easily
observable fact tends to weaken this point considerably: the same
person is often a speed freak, a pot-head, and an acid-head all at the
same time. Still, it is obvious that the responsible lawmakers and
opinion makers *ought* to be more concerned about the speed problem, and the question remains as to why they are not.

In 1961, at the same time as the passage of the *Narcotic Control
Act*, an amendment to the *Food and Drugs Act* created a new schedule of 'controlled drugs' made up of amphetamines and barbiturates. Under this amendment, trafficking in these drugs, or possession
for the purposes of trafficking, is punishable, upon summary conviction, to imprisonment for eighteen months, or upon conviction on
indictment, to ten years imprisonment. Simple possession is not a
criminal offence. However, the burden of proof, search and seizure,
and Writs of Assistance provisions described in regard to the *Narcotic Control Act* are substantially carried over into this category of
the *Food and Drugs Act*.[24] The police are hardly lacking in enforcement powers.

Early in 1969 the Canadian delegation at the United Nations
Narcotics Commission sponsored a resolution, which was unani-
mously adopted, calling for international controls on amphetamines
that follow "as closely as possible" the 1961 international convention regulating heroin, opium, cocaine, and other such 'hard' narcotics. The resolution was aimed at filling a gap prior to an international agreement covering amphetamine abuse.[25]

That some control will have to be exercised over the speed scene
is obvious. The simple fact is that the people most concerned are the

members of the drug subculture itself. Let us look at some examples from the underground press. In a recent article one writer suggested that methadrine

works directly on the cerebral cortex or the frontal lobes of the brain. The cortex itself suffers from chemical change and cellular death from lack of oxygen. Thus you have the back part of your memory beginning to fail. The heart muscles, the tonus of the peripheral blood vessels, kidney circulation and the gastrointestinal and urinary tracts are also affected . . .

The first stage of the starvation is the using up of body fats which appears as a loss of weight: your stomach and liver decrease in size; the linings of your intestines become smooth and thin, therefore becoming unable to absorb proteins, vitamins and other nutrients from any food. Later diarrhea ensues; women cease menstruating; men become impotent and lack sexual desire; your hair becomes dull and wiry; your scalp gets dry and scaly; your skin becomes dry and brittle; your teeth loosen and your gums bleed continually. In extreme cases cancrum oris can devour the tissues around your mouth, lips, and cheeks. Unfortunately, this is usually developed by younger people. Cirrhosis of the liver may also occur.[26]

Poet Allen Ginsberg has this to say:

Let's issue a general declaration to all the underground community, *contra speedamos ex cathedra*. Speed is anti-social, paranoid making, it's a drag, bad for your body, bad for your mind, in the long run uncreative . . . All the nice gentle dope fiends are getting screwed up by the real horror monster Frankenstein speedfreaks who are going around stealing and bad-mouthing everybody . . . The use of speed over two days tends to lead to irritability and insistency and a kind of Hitlerian fascist mentality . . . The junk problem is an easy problem to handle compared to the speed problem.[27]

Finally, William Burroughs, who has taken just about every drug there is to take, has this to say:

Pep pills and all variation of the benzedrine formulae present no valid excuse for continued existence . . . The whole spectrum of benzedrine intoxication is deplorable . . . Why not close the whole ugly scene once and for all by stopping the manufacture of benzedrine or any variation of the formula?[28]

It would seem that amphetamine abuse constitutes one of the gravest drug problems facing us at this moment. It is either physiologically addictive, or very close to it, with all the social problems that implies. But it is perhaps even worse than the opiates in two senses: first, it would seem to be physically more harmful to the user; second, its use seems to bring about personality changes that are more antisocial and unmanageable than those associated with opiate addiction. If it might be granted that the illegality of opiates has a major impact on the social role of the addict, it would not appear that the legal status of the speed freak has very much to do with his distasteful characteristics. If the opiate addict did not have to steal and engage in black market purchases, it is at least possible that he would no longer present the same threat to society that he is reputed to present now. But a speed freak who could buy all the methadrine he wanted at the corner drug store would still be a dangerous nuisance. In fact, the only difference might be that he would burn himself out even more quickly.

Solvent-inhalation – or glue-sniffing, as it is more popularly but less precisely known – is another practice that draws on the self-destructive urges lurking in the fever swamps of the human mind. But what sets solvent inhalation apart from all other forms of drug abuse is the age of the typical sniffer: the consistent pattern shows a mean age of about fourteen, in a range from eight to seventeen.[29] The reasons for this peculiar age specificity are not known. Some older youths do inhale solvents, but as a rule sniffing does not rival the use of cannabis, LSD, or amphetamines among older youths. In effect, solvent inhalation is a children's vice, and this fact presents very special problems to the lawmaker.

On October 10, 1968, Raymond Champagne (age ten) was found dead in an Ottawa park with a plastic bag over his head and empty tubes of glue scattered about the body. Raymond was only one of many such young victims, but the fact that his death occurred only a short distance from Parliament Hill brought the problem very close to home for the Federal government. Following this tragedy, an Ottawa newspaper sent out a young employee to purchase glue at various stories around the city; this was accomplished with no difficulty and at one store he was even advised to buy a cleaning fluid that would give a "better trip".[30]

Nitrous oxide and ether were among the first synthetic substances used for purposes of intoxication and hallucinogenic experiences. William James experimented with nitrous oxide in much the same way that present-day seekers after truth experiment with LSD. What nitrous oxide and ether have in common with the solvents inhaled by today's young children is the presence of volatile liquids that form solutions with lipids (fats and oils). Body cells contain lipids, and the vapors inhaled from volatile liquids readily dissolve in the lipids of the body cells. This would seem to be the basis of solvent intoxication, although the exact mechanism is not yet known.[31] Among the common household products containing volatile solvents are glues and cements (containing toluene and acetone); nail polish remover (acetone, alcohol, and aliphatic acetates); lighter fluid, cleaning fluid, and gasoline (naphtha, benzene, carbon tetrachloride); lacquer thinners (toluene and aliphatic acetates).[32] Toluene is the substance most commonly sought. The method of use is to squirt the solvent into a plastic bag and then insert the head into the bag and inhale the contents until the desired state of intoxication is reached. Euphoria, dizziness, and slurred speech are the immediate symptoms. Such mental confusions in young children are apt sometimes to lead to delusions of power and acts of violence and recklessness.[33] Hallucinations often occur, and perceptual distortions are common. If the inhalation continues too long, the anaesthetic effects become more predominant. Since the sniffer has his head enclosed in a plastic bag filled with rapidly hardening glue or cement, it is not difficult to see how asphyxia has often been the fate of sniffers who have lost consciousness.

Asphyxiation is only one of the dangers. Long-term physical and mental damage is probable, although not yet certain. Various symptoms arising from chronic use have been suggested in the medical literature, but the evidence is often conflicting and much more research needs to be done. Some deaths reported among solvent sniffers have been traced to lung disorders.[34] Recent research undertaken by the Addiction Research Foundation of Ontario found no brain damage among users, but did find liver abnormalities and, perhaps most serious of all, unusual breakage of chromosomes. Solvent sniffers showed six per cent chromosomal abnormalities compared to two per cent for the non-sniffers.[35] Physiological addiction has not been proved, but a strong psychological dependency is often created. Moreover, tolerance definitely develops, so that the amount of solvent required by a chronic sniffer far exceeds that required by the novice to achieve the same effects.

Sociologically, solvent sniffers appear to be underachievers with previous histories of delinquency. However, this finding is based on the sniffers known to authorities; they have usually come to notice because of antisocial behavior while under the influence of glue. It is not known whether better-adjusted children with better scholastic records also sniff solvents without demonstrating delinquent-type behavior. But even if the use of solvents only brings out tendencies already present, this can in itself be dangerous enough (witness alcohol). In 1967 a fifteen year old boy in Detroit raped and murdered two sisters, aged eight and six, who were on their way home from school. He was acquitted on the grounds that glue-sniffing had made the boy temporarily insane.[36]

Not surprisingly, parents have become quite concerned. The pressure on the Federal government to *do something* has become very strong. Unfortunately it is in just such panic situations that unwise legislation has often been brought into being. An inquest held into the death of Raymond Champagne recommended that the Criminal Code be amended to make it an offence to deliberately sniff solvents for the purposes of intoxication.[37] In 1967 a Juvenile Court judge refused to rule solvent sniffing an act of juvenile delinquency,[38] and the same view was upheld in the Alberta Supreme Court.[39] Later, however, a Toronto juvenile judge ruled that under s. 2(1)(h) of the *Juvenile Delinquents Act*, sniffing was a delinquent act, as the child was engaging in "sexual immorality or any similar form of vice".[40] The problem with all this is the same problem generated by all such punitive approaches: there is no evidence that it will work, and it will create a whole new class of criminals among the juvenile population. If one could muster more faith in our courts and correctional institutions as therapeutic agencies, one might be sympathetic to the use of the law to regulate personal behavior, but such faith is not easy to justify.

Another possible approach is through government regulation of the conditions of sale of dangerous solvents. Under new legislation covering hazardous products, the government will have the power to intervene actively in the production and sale of such products. The problem now becomes what to do with this power. It is curious to witness the touching faith that so many people seem to hold in the curative magic of Acts of Parliament. Toronto school trustee Alan Archer, backed by a 5,000 signature petition, asked the Minister of National Health and Welfare to have poison labels affixed to glue tubes and nail polish bottles, and to restrict sales of these articles to adults. Poison labels are hardly likely to deter any glue sniffer – he has probably been informed many times already that his habit is poisonous. Age restrictions are a farce. How many children who want to smoke cigarettes are really prevented by present laws? How many persons under twenty-one have been stopped from drinking alcohol when they really wanted to?

There is no possible way that the substances themselves can be banned. The products are all required for many legitimate purposes and at present the inclusion of volatile solvents is technologically necessary. More hopeful is the addition of nauseous odors or irritants to the products so as to make them too offensive for sniffing. Manufacturers have understandably been wary of this idea for fear of offending their regular customers, but the Testor Corporation of Canada Ltd. has recently developed an additive (volatile oil of mustard) for its brand of cement, which is not noticeable in normal use, but is definitely unpleasant when concentrated in a plastic bag – "like putting your nose clean into a fresh jar of horse radish and taking a deep breath." Testor has offered the formula to other manufacturers, and has suggested that it could be added to nail polish remover and wood cement as well.[41] If testing shows this additive to be effective, the government could make it mandatory.

Education is another weapon, but it is also, as Press and Done have suggested, a two-edged sword. It is possible that the more information is disseminated, the more children will find out about the practice and be enticed into it. The toxicity of solvent sniffing may be more apparent to the trained expert than to the child. The latter may, in fact, interpret warnings as 'scare' tactics on the part of generally untrustworthy adults.[42] Finally, we are left, as always, with the question of the drug user's motives. If parliament were able, by a stroke of the pen, to stop all volatile solvents from falling into the hands of children, some specific dangers to their health would have been removed; but how do we know that they would not simply turn to something else? It takes a lot of motivation to make a ten year old child sit with a vaporous bag over his head for hours breathing in fumes that would normally be considered unpleasant. What is it that can make a small child describe glue as her only friend? What ghastly deprivations must exist for such a statement to be possible? We hardly know how to begin answering such questions. But we had better start learning.

In an official statement the Ontario Addiction Research Foundation has suggested that

... legislation by itself is not an effective answer to this problem. Nor is education alone an effective answer. Treatment seems appropriate only in some cases; for example, where an underlying emotional disorder is the basis for the chronic abuse of various solvents. Research is clearly indicated ... While none of these approaches will suffice by itself, their combined application seems likely to be useful.[43]

To make matters worse, more and more household products are coming into use as intoxicants, continually increasing the chances of fatal accidents, and contributing to what must be a deepening sense of despair on the part of government officials who have to deal with the proliferating problems. Aerosol sprays of all kinds seem to be used for kicks. The United States Food and Drug Administration reported in May of 1969 that forty-two teen-agers had died inhaling the vapors from spray cans containing everything from mouth wash to cleaning fluid.[44] 'Frost-freaking' refers to breathing freon gas from glass-chillers. This apparently gives some hallucinogenic effects but it also freezes the larynx. In New York this practice has led to some deaths.[45] In October of 1968, a United States doctor reported that nasal sprays were making some people into "nasal medication addicts". Some sprays contain ethedrine, which could conceivably have hallucinogenic effects. Although at this time the Federal government was unaware of any such problem in Canada,[46] they did not have long to wait. Four months later a seventeen year old St. Catharines boy died fifteen minutes after inhaling a concentration of nasal spray in a handkerchief. It is not clear whether he died from an overdose of the medication or from the effects of freon, which was the propellant in the aerosol can.[47]

Even more bizarre types of drug use are practised here and there by adolescents as well as by some older drug users. There are reports of kids sitting in closed cars, spraying out the contents of insecticide cans, such as Raid, and breathing in the poisonous fumes. 'Orange juice freaks' inject orange juice into their arms. I have even been told that some antiwar demonstrators have freaked out on police tear gas! Anything is possible, and who knows what the future will hold by way of new drugs and new problems?

There is one last group of drugs that we should examine at this point. Barbiturates (sleeping pills) are quite probably among the most abused drugs we have with us today. But since barbiturate abuse tends to be concentrated among 'respectable' middle-class people, it attracts little attention. There is no doubt that barbiturates are physically addictive in much the same way as heroin: withdrawal symptoms are pronounced and prolonged.[48] Worse, the personality of the barbiturate addict tends to be far more offensive than that of the heroin addict. They tend to lose interest in their personal appearance, and to lose control over their emotional states. Barbiturate addiction is sometimes associated with opiate addiction. Barbiturates may be added to heroin on the black market, and the user may become addicted to both. Interestingly enough, at the Lexington treatment centre in Kentucky, some patients have been studied while under the influence of both opiates and barbiturates. With the former drugs they tend to be quiet, restrained, proficient at work and showing reduced sexuality. With barbiturates they tend to be confused in speech, stumbling in gait, obstinate, aggressive, and apt to masturbate in public.[49]

Even if not addicted, a barbiturate user is clearly a social menace behind the wheel of a car if he is under the immediate influence of the drug. Moreover, it is well known that many self-inflicted deaths are caused by barbiturates. Reports of Hollywood stars committing suicide with an overdose of sleeping pills are commonplace. In 1966 barbiturate poisoning was blamed for 167 of the 603 deaths in Ontario attributed to suicide. The chief of the Narcotics Control Branch of the Department of Health and Welfare has stated that barbiturates are "the most common cause associated directly or indirectly with deaths".[50] Barbiturates are included with amphetamines as 'controlled drugs' under the *Food and Drugs Act*, which means that simple possession is not an offence, although possession for the purpose of trafficking is an offence.[51]

Yet the public attitude toward the abuse of these drugs is curiously indifferent, rather like the attitude toward alcoholism, although lacking even the residue of prohibitionist moralism that still clings to alcohol use. The creation of the 'controlled drug' category was inspired by the fad in the 1950s among teen-agers for *goof-balls* (barbiturates, sometimes mixed with amphetamines). Today there does not seem to be much teen-age abuse of barbiturates, and so there is little public outcry. Doctors sometimes prescribe them for any sort of ailment for which there is no immediately identifiable cause: they calm hysterical patients down, and get them off the harried doctor's back. Anyone seriously interested in large scale consumption could probably get a number of prescriptions from different doctors. One cannot help wondering about the public outcry if long-haired hippies and rebellious high-school students were running a black market in barbiturates. But since it is mom and dad who reach for the sleeping pills every night, there is only public complacency. That such complacency also spells hypocrisy seems to bother the public not at all.

Footnotes

[1]Michael Valpy, "Official LSD paper is adopted by users," *Globe and Mail* (April 30, 1969).

[2]S. H. Snyder *et al*, "DOM(STP), a new hallucinogenic drug, and DOET: effects in normal subjects," *American Journal of Psychiatry*, vol. 125, no. 3 (Sept., 1968), pp. 358-64.

[3]"STP formula reported taken from Dow firm," *Globe and Mail* (Aug. 4, 1967).

[4]See K. R. Capper, "Lysergic Acid Derivitives in Morning Glory seeds," in C. W. M. Wilson, ed., *The Pharmacological and Epidemiological Aspects of Adolescent Drug Dependence* (Oxford, Pergamon Press, 1968), pp. 75-82.

[5]Sidney Cohen, *The Beyond Within: the LSD Story*, 2nd ed. (New York, Atheneum, 1967), p. 20.

[6]J. Robertson Unwin, "Illicit Drug Use Among Canadian Youth," part I, *Canadian Medical Association Journal*, vol. 98 (Feb. 24, 1968).

[7]Richard Evans Schultes, "Hallucinogens of Plant Origin," *Science*, vol. 163 (Jan. 17, 1969), p. 252.

[8]Norman R. Farnsworth, "Hallucinogenic Plants," *Science*, vol. 162 (Dec. 6, 1968).

[9]J. S. Slotkin, *The Peyote Religion* (Glencoe, Illinois, The Free Press, 1956).

[10]R. E. L. Masters and Jean Houston, *The Varieties of Psychedelic Experience* (New York, Delta Books, 1967), p. 47.

[11]Schultes, *op. cit.*

[12]Carlos Castenada, *The Teachings of Don Juan: A Yaqui Way of Knowledge* (New York, Ballantine, 1969), contains fascinating remarks on datura.

[13]"Coroner wants drug removed from shelf," *Globe and Mail* (Jan. 5, 1968).

[14]Unwin, *op. cit.*

[15]Aldous Huxley, *The Devils of Loudon: a Study in the Psychology of Power Politics and Mystical Religion in the France of Cardinal Richelieu* (New York, Harper and Row, 1952), pp. 313-15.

[16]Castenada, *op. cit.* Of all the personal accounts of hallucinogenic experiences, Castenada's is both the most bewildering and the most thought-provoking.

[17]Paul and Percival Goodman, *Communitas: Means of Livelihood and Ways of Life* (New York, Random House, 1947), pp. 149-50.

[18]Alan W. Watts, *The Joyous Cosmology: Adventures in the Chemistry of Consciousness* (New York, Random House, 1962), pp. 86-88.

[19]Oriana Josseau Kalant, *The Amphetamines: Toxicity and Addiction*. Brookside Menograph No. 5. Published for the Alcoholism and Drug Addiction Research Foundation of Ontario, (Toronto, University of Toronto Press, 1966), p. 133.

[20]J. C. Kramer, V. S. Fischman, D. C. Littlefield, *Journal of the American Medical Association*, vol. 201 (1967), p. 305.

[21]Unwin, *op. cit.*

[22]Kramer *et al, op. cit.*

[23]"Tore off man's foot, gets two years in jail," *Globe and Mail* (Feb. 2, 1968).

[24]9-10 Elizabeth II (1961) c. 37.

[25]"UN classified amphetamines with heroin," *Globe and Mail* (Jan. 29, 1969).

[26]Danny Biscope, "Speed," *Octopus*, vol. 2, no. 8 (April 14, 1969).

[27]*Canadian Free Press* (July 5-19, 1968).

[28]William Burroughs, "Academy 23: a Deconditioning," *The Village Voice* (July 6, 1967), p. 21.

[29]Andrew I. Malcolm, "Solvent-sniffing and its Effects," *Addictions*, vol. 15, no. 2 (Summer, 1968), p. 20.

[30]Mike McDermott, "No questions asked — and you can even buy a complete 'trip kit'," *Ottawa Citizen* (Oct. 12, 1968).

[31]Malcolm, *op. cit.*, pp. 13-14.

[32]Unwin, *op. cit.*, p. 403.

[33]Edward Press and Alan K. Done, "Solvent Sniffing," *Pediatrics*, vol. 39, nos. 3 and 4 (March and April, 1967).

[34]Unwin, *loc. cit.*

[35]Joan Hollobon, "Find broken chromosomes in glue-sniffers," *Globe and Mail* (Feb. 26, 1969).

[36]"Glue to blame, boy acquitted of 2 murders," *Globe and Mail* (Aug. 17, 1967).

[37]David Smithers, "Glue sniffing," *Ottawa Citizen* (Dec. 18, 1968).

[38]"Glue sniffing not a crime; boy freed," *Globe and Mail* (July 5, 1967).

[39]*R. v. Pandiak* (1967) 61 W.W.R. 207.

[40]Graham Parker, "Glue sniffing," *Criminal Law Quarterly*, vol. 11, no. 2 (Feb., 1969).

[41]Betty Lee, "Additive puts punch in glue," *Globe and Mail* (April 10, 1969). "To save young lives" (Editorial), *Globe and Mail* (April 11, 1969).

[42]Press and Done, *op. cit.*

[43]*Approaches to the Control of Glue sniffing*, Statement from the Alcoholism and Drug Addiction Research Foundation (Jan. 18, 1968).

[44]"Mouthwash 'sniffing' kills 42," *Ottawa Citizen* (May 9, 1969).

[45]*New York Times* (Oct. 4, 1967).

[46]"Nose drop danger," *Ottawa Citizen* (Oct. 16, 1968).

[47]"St. Catharines youth, 17, died after inhaling vapors of a cold medication, coroner says," *Globe and Mail* (Feb. 11, 1969).

[48]Robert S. DeRopp, *Drugs and the Mind* (New York, Grove Press, 1961), p. 163.

[49]Peter Laurie, *Drugs: Medical, Psychological, and Social Facts* (Harmondsworth, Middlesex, Penguin Books, 1967), p. 63.

[50]"Drugs termed problem with wives, businessmen," *Globe and Mail* (Aug. 24, 1967).

[51]9-10 Elizabeth II (1961), c. 37. Amended by P.C. 1962-1471 (Oct. 18, 1962), and 17-18 Elizabeth II (1969), c. 41, ss. 7-8.

Drugs, Youth, and Education

One of those strangely elusive but compelling myths that echo down the generations and centuries is that of the Pied Piper of Hamelin, whose music stole all the children of the town away from their parents and into a mountain, never to return. The recurrence of this story suggests that it holds a certain fascination that goes beyond the appeal of the merely quaint or curious legend. A great deal of emphasis has been recently laid on the difficulties of adolescence and on the alleged deviations and abnormalities of the adolescent who cannot quite bear the strains of growing up. Perhaps too little emphasis has been laid on the difficulties of parenthood and deep psychological strains that accompany the raising of children. At best parenthood is an ambivalent condition: on the one hand, people yearn for immortality and the perpetuation of oneself in a newborn infant is, in a symbolic sense at the least, a continuance of one's own being; on the other hand, a child is an altogether different creature than oneself, capable of continual and apparently independent change. The story of the Pied Piper embodies this ambivalence perfectly. The parents and their political representatives brought the trouble on their own heads by refusing to pay the Piper for clearing the town of rats. In revenge the Piper played a tune that irresistably drew all the children behind him. The parents were unable to persuade the Piper to stop nor could they stop their children. And thus their own flesh and blood, those tiny reflections of themselves were drawn out of their power and severed from their source forever.

The Pied Piper myth serves to explain the trauma of children leaving the home by means of that familiar old *deus ex machina*, the Outside Agitator. The children, one might assume, would otherwise have grown up in close emulation of their beloved parents were it not for that Outside Agitator and his strange music. And so, instead of trying to understand *why* their children were different and *why* they wanted to go their own way, the Outside Agitator could be blamed, and any guilt feelings on the part of the parents thus could be easily suppressed; in our own day, no doubt, various parliamentary notables would demand that immigration officials not allow any more such Agitators into the country.

The great drug scare is in a sense a modern re-enactment of the Pied Piper story. Overrun with stress, anxiety and confusion – just as Hamelin was overrun with rats – respectable middle-class society called in not the Pied Piper, but the Pill Pusher, and artificially dispelled its troubles with aspirins, tranquilizers, stimulants, and barbiturates, as well as alcohol and tobacco. But soon their own children began to grow threateningly different. Boys grew long 'effeminate' hair; girls shamelessly wore miniskirts. Across a wide and frightening spectrum, from religion to politics, from clothes to music, from peace demonstrations to student protests, from attitudes toward work to attitudes toward sex, *something* has obviously been happening. How many hard-working, God-fearing, tax-paying, right-thinking, middle-aged, middle-class parents have not confronted the terrible thought that they have raised a generation of monsters who threaten to turn on their progenitors and destroy all that they hold dear? But of course it is all the fault of the Pied Piper. Above all we must never admit that the changes that have taken place are the result of the separate individuality of young people and of their conscious choice. Behavior should be normal and predictable like that of mice in a cage. Stimulus: response. Cause: effect. When the simple and reassuring equations break down, when dramatic and bizarre changes in behavior occur, then the blame must be laid on some Machiavellian outside force. Marijuana . . . LSD . . . Timothy Leary . . . Jerry Rubin . . . The Rolling Stones . . . all these become candidates for the role of the Pied Piper.

The problem with the Pied Piper theory, however, is that it really does not explain anything at all. Why, after all, did the Piper have such a compelling hold on all the children of Hamelin? Why were the adults not drawn irresistibly in his wake as well? If their children were not already different why were they alone attracted to the Piper's tune? *What was it in the Piper's strange music that only the children could hear?*

To assert that young people taking drugs are merely blank slates upon which some chemical substance has sketched a personality is a point of view as insulting in its implications as it is oblivious to reality. The Celts believed that when one became drunk on ale one was no longer oneself but was in the possession of a deity. It nevertheless seems unlikely that they went so far as to attribute all the ale-drinker's subsequent behavior to the influence of the deity. Any attempt at explaining why young people take drugs had best start by rejecting outright a modern reversion to animism. Just because some of the wilder elements among the drug cultists have drifted into referring to LSD as God does not mean that less bemused heads need accept such an essentially idiotic fallacy.

People tend to eat because they are hungry, drink because they are thirsty, and make love because they feel desire. It is at least equally probable that they take drugs that alter their consciousness because they want their consciousness to be changed. This is a relatively simple premise, but many people seem highly resistant to accepting even the most elementary implications of individual free will, especially when applied to young people. In the 1930s marijuana was referred to as the "assassin of youth" – a phrase coined by Mr. Anslinger of the U.S. Narcotics Bureau – and posters warned that within it lurked MURDER! INSANITY! DEATH! Thankfully even the enemies of drug use have gained in sophistication since those days, but a variation of the Pied Piper myth is still current. As one Member of Parliament recently explained to the House of Commons, any liberalization of the laws dealing with marijuana would only benefit "the behind the scenes peddlers working on behalf of the international crime syndicates for whom the illegal distribution of drugs brings in many millions of dollars annually, and who in pursuit of financial returns do not hesitate to destroy a whole generation of young people."[1] The truth is much less garish, but perhaps even more unsettling to those who refuse to recognize young people as autonomous, self-governing human beings. The truth is that the Vancouver teen-ager with pot carefully stashed away in an envelope probably got it from another teen-ager who got it from another, etc., eventually leading to a student who smuggled it across the Mexican border into California inside the tires of his car. The Toronto teen-ager pasing out hashish at a party may have got it from a friend in Ottawa who received it in the mail from another friend travelling in North Africa or in India.

If we are ever going to come to grips with the reasons why young people take drugs, we must at least grant that they are responding to needs that precede and are of more fundamental importance than drug use itself. In other words there are problems, some old, some new, to which drugs are an attempted solution.

Before going any further, two points should be made clear. In what follows I am merely setting down some impressions, backed neither by scientific studies nor by learned authorities. Secondly, any generalizations should be taken as having less than universal applicability: young people are as diverse and as divided among themselves as older people.

We might begin by making one necessary distinction between leaders and followers. There are always going to be some kids who have no very clear objective with regard to drugs but who will either follow the crowd or will try to emulate those who are generally admired. It is this category that probably swells the statistics on youthful drug use that the media like to brandish, but it is most likely that such impressionable types are more preponderant among those who have tried various drugs once or twice than among the regular users. Since the first experience with marijuana is usually disappointing and since any experience with LSD can be unsettling in the extreme, a certain amount of motivation is required to persevere. There is in fact a considerable drop-out rate among would-be drug users. Less emphasis should be put on surveys that ask "have you ever smoked pot?" and more on surveys designed to find out how many use drugs *regularly*. It would seem to me that only the exceptionally weak-willed person will continue to ingest something as risky as an illegal drug unless it answers some need more profound than merely going along with friends.

Among those who willfully persist, I think we can delineate three main groups: Escapists, Explorers, and Rebels. Let us examine each of these in turn.

Escapists. As long as humanity has existed people have tried to escape an unpleasant or painful reality by chemically altering their consciousness. For generations now in North America, disturbed young people from slum areas have become addicted to opiates. So long as there are people who cannot cope with the world there will probably be some who will seek the twilight oblivion of the junkie's paradise. No doubt those young people who live in depressed urban slums will continue to be susceptible to heroin's appeals. While teen-agers and college students have been experimenting with opium here and there, this seems to rest more on opium's reputation as an exotic oriental practice than on its connection with heroin and morphine. It would be foolish to deny that the latter drugs may have made some slight headway among groups, who until recently would have had no ready access to them, but the RCMP's strictures aside, opiate addiction does not seem to be a very important new threat outside its traditional areas of prevalence.

Opiates are, however, not the only drugs of escape. Glue-sniffing, pot-smoking, and even acid-dropping can be used primarily as ways of escaping. *Turning-on* can just as well mean *turning-off* and one of the very real dangers of marijuana, and particularly of the more potent hashish, is the tendency of the chronic user to simply float downstream and let the world go to Hell. In general the Escapists are more numerous among the hard-core drop-out crowd – commonly known as *hippies*, a title that in the hands of the media means next to nothing – than among students, whether at the high-school or the college level. The reason for this is not hard to find: anyone who really sets his mind to pursuing escape is not likely to last very long at an educational institution. Whether he drops out or is dropped out is a mere matter of detail. It is among the Escapists that the greatest dangers of drug dependency exist. Whether or not the substance leads to physical signs of addiction or merely to psychological habituation may not be very important. More important is that an individual primarily interested in escape will very likely become involved, to an unhealthy and perhaps self-destructive extent, with the drug that offers such escape.

Explorers. In sharp antithesis to the motives of the Escapists there are many young people who use drugs to search out new experiences, to test the limits of their senses and of their understanding. But even among the Explorers themselves there can be detected two quite divergent tendencies, one of which is reckless but in many ways admirable, the other of which is crude and wholly self-destructive.

To take the latter type first there have always been adolescents out for kicks – which may mean anything from driving at 100 miles per hour in a 35 mile zone to vandalism to gang rapes. The current archetype of this personality is the Hell's Angel motorcycle outlaw and his various imitators in Canada, such as the Satan's Choice gang. If nothing else the motorcycle gangs at least have achieved a certain style and *panache* in their violence; not even that much can be said for the less distinguished *greasers* who hate hippies and students as much as they hate straight society. Alcohol is probably the most common and best-loved drug among these ranks – although there is no deep prejudice against others, such as barbiturates, which as *goof-balls* had a wave of popularity in the 1950s. Speed may now be the most popular drug next to alcohol among this group: it certainly fits within their philosophy and life-style.

Not only the greasers but also many more respectable-looking teen-agers may use drugs for simple thrill-seeking reasons. Young people are just as often *bored* as they are alienated. Not allowed to become full-fledged members of adult society but no longer children, adolescents may often find themselves caught up in the middle of an idle and endlessly empty life. Anything to break the dull monotony is welcomed, especially if it is something that gives the uncertain young male a chance to show his virility (which, true to the dominant values of our society, is usually taken to mean aggression and physical courage). This involves playing with death; perhaps screaming around a curve on a motorcycle at an insane speed and hanging in there all the way around, tasting the presence of death in the air; or perhaps shooting amphetamines directly into the veins and to hell with those warnings that *Speed Kills*. Needless to say, education campaigns that stress the personal dangers of drug abuse will be about as effective in discouraging this type of user as atrocity pictures from Vietnam would be in turning a sadist against the war.

There is, however, another aspect of the Explorer category that does not have the same openly self destructive bent. There are a growing number of young people who are genuinely searching for an understanding of who and what they are. To them the old answers have proved inadequate, if not meaningless, and thus new methods of exploration have to be devised. It is impossible to underestimate the trauma of growing up in a world where there no longer even seems to be an accepted definition of what man *is* and what his place is in the universe. The sensitive and thoughtful young person confronts a philosophical and moral abyss. And as Friedrich Nietzsche remarked, "if you gaze long into an abyss, the abyss will gaze back into you."[2] Against that awful potentiality there is much desperate testing of the limits of the human personality, much striving to redefine the meaning of human existence. This no doubt sounds overblown and pretentious, but there is no denying the intensity of the struggle going on within many troubled young minds. The point is that very little can any longer be taken for granted and in such a world the most immediate questions are also the most fundamental. Hallucinogenic drugs are a raft upon which one may set out to explore the uncharted inner seas of the mind, a key that opens the door of an old but vast room long forgotten by bustling, self-confident science and rationalism. For the reasons already touched upon in discussing LSD, it is the non-rational, mystical, ecstatic realms of human experience that are most likely to be explored by contemporary seekers of truth, and the place of drugs in such a search is obvious.

Another factor that enters into this scene is the existential quality of youthful questing. It is now obvious even to reactionary moralists that traditional moral authority is in an advanced stage of decay. I personally doubt that any recrudescence of the dying *corpus* is now possible, but in any event it is a fact that among young people more and more importance is being placed on the radical necessity of individual choice in concrete situations, rather than on the wholesale acceptance of an abstract ethical code to be applied indiscriminately to any and all situations. It is the failure to account for this altered moral perspective that helps explain the failure of the law to control drug use among youth. The old edict that sex is only moral if it occurs between duly married couples is being replaced by the idea that what is truly important is the attitude of the personalities involved regardless of external social judgments. Similarly the idea that taking a certain drug is always and in any conceivable circumstances wrong is being replaced by the notion that it all depends on the motives of the person involved, which may be reprehensible but may just as well be admirable.

Rebels. Implicit in the description of both the Escapists and the Explorers has been the aura of rebellion. To a certain extent one may speak of a third distinct group of drug takers among whom rebelliousness itself seems to be the prime motive. First of all there is the simple desire to be different from the adult society. It is no accident that long-hair, miniskirts, rock music, and 'free' schools have been matched by the evolution of distinctive intoxicants. It would be altogether too much to expect that Rebels striving zealously to declare their independence from their parents' way of life should be content to get together on Saturday night and pour out a gin-and-tonic or a Scotch-and-soda. This rebelliousness presents the law-maker with a bizarre situation. Some kids smoke pot, not because they like it very much, but simply as a protest against what is seen as an unjust and intolerable law; many smoke it simply because it is forbidden fruit. If marijuana were allowed to be used openly, there might well be a shift of the Rebel group into some different, but still illegal, drug. This parallels the attitude of a girl who once told me that the New Morality could ruin sex by making it appear no longer a sin! Doubtless there are deep psychological roots to the feeling that pleasure can only come from the violation of a taboo, but I must confess that this viewpoint leaves me somewhat baffled. Any well-intentioned reformer, it seems, must be prepared to allow for a cer-tain degree of sheer human perversity when trying to bring about a more humane legal situation.

The Rebel mentality has its more positive aspects, however, and here too drugs have a certain place. Alcohol is increasingly seen as a symbol of the rough, aggressive, competitive capitalist system from which the young Rebel – or to be more precise, the young middle-class Rebel – wishes to be emancipated. Many see marijuana, by con-trast, as the symbol of more peaceful, communal, and loving form of social relationships. Passing the joint or the hookah around from person to person recalls the half-forgotten social rituals of the pre-industrial past. Perhaps McLuhan's concepts of the Global Vil-lage and the new tribalism have here generated an almost literal response. What is important is to recognize that pot and acid are felt to be *one* means of opening people to an understanding of one another. They have never been thought of as the *only* way. It was left to the orthodox media to assert that every time a rock group makes a reference to 'love' it is really making a leering reference to drugs. *Honi soit qui mal y pense.*

There is also a rebellion of the young against technology. Some kids explain the use of LSD as being their own personal revolt against the dehumanization and depersonalization of a technological world through the deliberate invocation of mystical or primitivist states of mind. In effect they are consciously folding, stapling, bending, tearing, (and perhaps mutilating?) themselves so that the relentless Social Computer will not be able to sort and process them. This is a desire for which an increasing number of people today might express a certain amount of secret admiration, but nowhere among youthful aspirations does one find a greater ambivalence than on this point. In a very real sense today's young are the children of technology. Television, films, radio, cars, motorcycles, airplanes – all these are the womb in which today's youth were shaped. And it is not without a certain irony that one notes that a revolt against the domination of science and technology is based upon yet another gimmick, a synthetic drug. A revitalized Luddite attack on the machinery of our artificial world will have to await more whole-hearted recruits than the consumers of Lysergic Acid Diethylamide.

I have touched on some of the reasons why young people use drugs. There are no doubt many more reasons than the ones I have enumerated. Obviously there are a wide variety of motives at work; the point is to avoid the fallacy that the simple act of taking an illegal drug is necessarily a more important fact than all the underlying factors that led up to drug use. To someone who suffers an extreme psychotic reaction to an LSD experience, the taking of the drug may in itself be of grave importance; to another individual who smokes pot occasionally with friends, drug use may in itself mean next to nothing, scarcely more than an after-dinner liqueur or a good cigar. The young glue sniffer may seem to be in a sorry plight but how many of his real troubles would be removed by keeping glue out of his hands? A further point to be made is that kids who use drugs usually have reasons for doing so. They may have good reasons or bad reasons, their ideas may be delusive, and sometimes the motives may even be quite evidently self-destructive, but their actions are more often than not deliberate, and they must be dealt with as such.

This leads us to the question of education, which is being looked upon increasingly by Canadian authorities as a possible solution to the problems of drug abuse. *Education* has long been a liberal panacea for all social ills just as *discipline* has been the conservative alternative. But before examining either education or discipline we must first examine the thorny problem of authority and what it means both for those on the giving and those on the receiving end. The question of what constitutes authority is of course a complex problem, much debated by political philosophers, which hardly lends itself to the brief consideration we can give it here. But at the risk of oversimplification I should like to put forward an hypothesis, upon which we might proceed.

When someone issues a command or puts forward a point of view that is considered *authoritative*, the content of the message is accepted primarily because of the *source* from which it comes. That is to say, it is assumed that such a message is backed by superior knowledge or wisdom or moral goodness because the sender is believed or reputed to hold such knowledge, wisdom or goodness. Once, however, that some rational explanation of the message is demanded, then at that moment the pure authority relationship beings to break down, since the messages are no longer being accepted at their face value on the authority of their source. If explanations are provided and accepted, it is not authority as such but *persuasion* that is at work, since the explanation will presumably be based on facts or logic which are themselves independent of the person giving the explanation. In a tradition-directed society, for example, certain persons possess inherent authority based perhaps on heredity or on the position they hold (priest, king, etc.). Such persons are not expected to explain the content of authoritative messages, nor are others expected to demand explanations, but only to behave in the manner indicated. When explanations are demanded, persons in positions of authority have a choice: they may provide such explanations, which, whether accepted or not accepted, tend to destroy traditional authority; or they may choose to enforce their authority by means of the coercive *power* at their command. In the latter case there is no longer any concern with the individual's inner assent or dissent – all that matters is his outward compliance. Conservatism then can have two quite separate faces: it can rationally or reasonably explain why an institution or a policy should be maintained in the face of criticism; or it may simply threaten critics with force. But in neither case is the traditional concept of authority retained. Traditional authority can be maintained only so long as the revolutionary question "why?" is not asked, or at least is not widely asked.

All this is important because there is, I believe, convincing evidence that we are now entering a period when radical criticism is being applied to traditional authority in matters of personal morality, in much the same way that radical criticism was applied to traditional political authority in the years leading up to the French Revolution. What is essential in such a situation is to recognize that persuasion alone is likely to have an effect. Traditional authority is inoperative at best, and at worst a laughing-stock. When this happens, the response of bewildered conservatives is to restore 'order' by means of imposing discipline externally. Yet how far this solution is from the original conservative ideal of inner assent to the moral order of society can be glimpsed in the blustering vehemence and the uneasy rationalizations with which punitive prison sentences are handed down in our courts against young drug users.

In Manitoba in 1968, a twenty year old boy was sentenced by a magistrate to one month in jail and a $400 fine on a marijuana charge. The reason given by the magistrate for the relatively light sentence was that the accused had discontinued drug use, and the magistrate did not wish to jeopardize his university studies. The Federal Justice Department appealed the decision and asked the Manitoba Court of Appeal to impose a stiffer sentence. The Court of Appeal agreed and raised the sentence to one year. In the opinion of the Court, the magistrate had "seemed much too concerned with the possible rehabilitation of this young offender and by the fact that a long term of incarceration would deny him access to the university this fall. In doing so he completely disregarded the interests of the community and put those of the individual ahead of the community."[3]

This same theory of 'deterrence' as the prime responsibility of the political and judicial system in meeting drug use was stated in a somewhat similar marijuana case in British Columbia, involving a university student, where a suspended sentence imposed by a magistrate was changed to one of six months imprisonment by the provincial Court of Appeal.[4] In this decision the point was made that middle-class offenders ought to be subject to the same punishment as working-class offenders, but the inconsistency of this argument was revealed by an editorial in the *Criminal Law Quarterly*, which noted that the same Court in the previous year had sentenced two middle-class businessmen convicted of stealing $20,000 from the B.C. Hydro Authority to only one month in jail and a $1,000 fine.[5] As the *Quarterly* suggests: "not everyone smokes marijuana, but everyone cheats the Government in some way, and the Court had an excellent opportunity to deter generally. In that case, the British Columbia Court of Appeal made very clear that retribution has no place in the law."[6] To the old complaint that there is one law for the rich and another for the poor can be added a new suggestion, that there is one law for the old and another for the young. This is not to suggest that some sort of baleful malevolence has gained the upper hand in the administration of justice but it is to suggest that traditional moral authority on such matters is now undergoing the hideous convulsions of a prolonged and painful death, and that its place has slowly, often imperceptibly, been taken over by the exercise of naked power, by the enforcement of external discipline, and the practice of making examples of those unlucky enough to be caught – "*pour encourager les autres*," as Voltaire explained the execution of Admiral Byng.

The difficulty is that however often the ritual incantation of the magic phrase *law and order* is repeated, *law* and *order* continue to be quite separate and sometimes antithetical concepts. When the exercise of law is seen as unjust, individuals who are made examples usually end up by being examples not of the wrongness of their personal actions but of the tyranny of the system that makes them into martyrs. Too much *law* of this kind leads not to *order* but to *disorder*, to angry defiance, protest, and greater solidarity among the groups who most feel the weight of the law.

An eighteen year old girl is before a Toronto court, charged with selling ten dollars worth of marijuana to an undercover RCMP agent. She is addressed by the Judge in the following terms: "You are a dope pusher and an addict . . . You were engaged in a vile, dirty, profitable business – you were destroying other people."[7] Does anyone who has any understanding of youth and knows anything about drugs, seriously believe that such a statement will elicit any response other than contempt?

An Ontario County Judge is sentencing a nineteen year old boy to a year and a half for trafficking in marijuana: "You, along with many like you, pay too much attention to publicity-seeking, misguided persons who seem to think that first offenders in these trafficking cases should be given suspended sentences. I might say that first offenders had better not find themselves in this court."[8] Thus it is not just those who break the law who fall under judicial displeasure but even those who advocate a change in the law. It may be noted in passing that the Judge's condemnation would even include public statements made by the Minister of National Health and Welfare, but the implications are nevertheless disturbing. In England a major newspaper and a former Conservative cabinet minister[9] have publicly stated that freedom of speech ought not to extend to those who would advocate changes in the drug laws. And in Canada we have the example of the Senate seriously considering making "promotion" of the use of LSD a criminal offence, "promotion" to be defined by the Governor in Council. When force and deterrence are adopted as the leading policies, this is the road upon which we set out. We ought to take a long, long look down that road before we begin.

After tasting the rather bitter brew of repression, the Federal government, as well as some provincial governments, now seems more interested in tempering power with persuasion. Partly this is due to hardy (perhaps foolhardy) resistance on the part of youth. A special Crown prosecutor in narcotics cases in Ottawa, who had previously pressed for stiff sentences, recently showed commendable courage and honesty in admitting to a public meeting in the city that the theory of deterrence had not worked, and should be de-emphasized in favor of another approach.[10]

Despite the decent, liberal ring to the word *education*, just how effective can education be in dealing with drug use? I think it can be said with a fair degree of certainty that if the aim of education is taken to be the elimination of all youthful drug use, then education is bound to be a failure. A second point to be made is that if education is understood as being a disguised form of hierarchical authority, a one-way system of communication, a method of control, rather than an exchange of ideas or a cooperative search for meaning, then education will meet the same fate as deterrence – it will be neither admired nor respected. If anyone thinks that education can be an assembly-line stamping of moral imperatives on youth like the stamping of company labels on a line of bottles, then they might as well forget about it and start considering something more sensible, like burning drug-users at the stake, or lopping off their hands. Education at its best can, however, create a type of authority, where the authority is based not on power but on the respect that is granted to greater knowledge and wisdom. But the difficulties of arriving at this ideal situation are enormous. Let us take an impressionistic look at some of the parameters of the problem.

Radio report: A U.S. government official, addressing *Toc Alpha* (a youth group promoting temperance) in Ontario said that no changes should be allowed in laws against marijuana; even if it were not physically addictive, he said, it was psychologically habituating. The speaker went on to criticize *Toc Alpha* for attempting to stop the sale of alcoholic beverages in the hotel where the meeting was held. "You must face the fact," he said, "that we live in an alcohol culture."

Press report: "Careless smoking by intoxicated persons was blamed yesterday by a coroner's jury investigating the deaths of three persons in a fire . . . 'You have here people, alcohol, and cigarets, and there is no law against alcohol or cigarets', the Coroner said."[11]

The Senate of Canada: Senator Hartland Molson (President, Molson Breweries), during a debate on LSD: "[Timothy] Leary has built himself a little empire. He has hundreds of thousands of the young worshipping at his feet. He is a vicious man. He is a wicked man. As a matter of fact, anything that could be done to Leary would not be enough. I believe that type of person has no place at large in our society . . . We do not want him around."[12]

Robert de Ropp, biochemist: "Alcohol passes rapidly into the blood stream and is quickly distributed to every organ in the body . . . Signs of intoxication begin to be seen as soon as the alcohol has entered the brain. First comes the inhibition of the function of the cerebral cortex produced by a drink of two to three ounces of whisky and corresponding to 0.05 per cent of alcohol in the blood . . . When the concentration of alcohol in the blood rises to about .1 per cent the depressant influence spreads to those centers in the brain which regulate movements . . . At a concentration of .2 per cent of alcohol in the blood the entire motor area of the brain is affected and the depressant effect of the drug spreads to those centers in the midbrain which control the emotional manifestations of men . . . With .3 per cent of alcohol in his blood the drinker's brain becomes affected in that area which is concerned with sensory perception . . . At a level of .4 per cent or .5 per cent in the blood, alcohol depresses the whole perception area in the brain and the drinker becomes comatose. Finally, with .6 per cent to .7 per cent of alcohol in the blood, our drinker dies a swift and painless death, his breathing and the beating of his heart arrested by paralysis of the centers that control these vital functions."[13]

Magazine article: ". . . To the medical scientists now studying the effects of LSD on the human body, the three letters invoke a threat of deadly damage now and appalling defects for generations yet unborn . . . The new research, begun only this year, is unfolding one horror after another before it is even out of the preliminary stages."[14]

Medical journal: "It seems that the time has come when women should be told frankly that if they smoke [tobacco] they not only put their own lives in jeopardy, but if they continue to do so during pregnancy, also expose their unborn infants to an unnecessary risk."[15]

Press report: "A raging controversy over marijuana and LSD in Britain took a bizarre turn yesterday with a report that a law graduate drilled a hole in his head while under the influence of marijuana."[16]

Press report: "Sperm banks should be set up for spacemen because prolonged exposure to weightlessness might damage the chromosomes in astronaut's sex cells and result in the conception of defective children. This suggestion comes from two scientists who have discovered unusually high rates of chromosome damage in the sperm cells of fruit flies that orbited earth in unmanned biological satellites."[17]

Press report: "Dr. Norman Yoder, the Pennsylvania state official who falsely reported six college students were blinded while under the influence of the drug LSD, will not be prosecuted by the state."[18]

World Health Organization report: Heart disease accounted for almost one-third of all deaths in Western nations in 1964. It was felt that this high incidence reflected the stress which the fast-paced, competitive way of life places on the individual. Suicide continued to increase in the industrialized nations.

RCMP Commissioner: "The lawless 'beat' generation will create a mounting fear of anarchy in Canada unless it is met firmly by police with 'massive public and governmental support'."[19]

Whiskey advertisement: DON'T GULP.
> Soft whiskey
> goes down so nice and natural,
> you might be tempted to.
> Don't. It's real 86 proof stuff.

U.S. Senate hearing: "John Steinbeck IV, son of the author, told a Senate subcommittee today American youth considers the major health hazard of the day to be the military draft, not marijuana. 'If you smoke marijuana, you're going to wake up tomorrow', he said, while the draft leads to 'death for a vast number of the nation's youth'."[20]

Oakville, Ontario, Conference on Youth: "A psychopharmacologist with the Ontario Hospital in Toronto, told the conference that a drug education movie shown in Toronto schools 'and put out by the police with the assistance of the schools' contained eleven glaring errors of fact. Asked 'how dangerous is marijuana?', the director of the drug research project at the Queen Street clinic, answered that he didn't know enough about marijuana to answer the question. He said there had been no significant research on marijuana since 1946 ... After the conference, one long-haired, bearded youth wearing granny spectacles surprised reporters by quoting from the last major marijuana study in 1946. He had long ago read the report. It seems obvious that some youths have very thoroughly done their homework on marijuana – much more than many of the parents who admonish and lecture them on the evils of drugs."[21]

What does all this mean? If you are asking yourself this question after reading the last few paragraphs you will have grasped the precise point I am trying to make. The individual is bombarded with information from all sides and through all media. Some of this information is sound and useful, some is dubious, some is misleading, some is asinine. In the more optimistic nineteenth century, Jeremy Bentham could suggest that if the chemical composition of medicines were required to be printed on the bottles then quack remedies would fail to find a market. What Bentham might have thought of people who will eat, drink, swallow, smoke, sniff or inject any substance put into their hands is best left to the imagination. But even for those somewhat more discriminating, the search for meaningful and reliable information is frustrating and confusing and often hopeless. The revolution in medical science and technology has spawned a nightmare world of chemical incomprehension, a landscape filled with thousands and thousands of drugs with mystifying names and unknown functions. Every year people consume tons of acetylsalicylic acid (aspirin), yet only now, years after it has become as much a part of the ordinary household as roast beef and apple pie, are some of its bad side-effects becoming known. Who can tell? After observing the passing fads in wonder drugs and the various passing drug scares that flare up from time to time in the press, I have taken it as a sound working principle that any drug thought of as a cure-all is almost certain to be later exposed as causing anything from cancer to pimples, probably within a decade of its original fad. The only sensible approach to such a situation is to refuse all chemical invasions entirely but even this solution is only possible by retreating to the mountains, for the urban water supply is chlorinated and fluoridated and the urban air that we breathe in any major Canadian city is polluted with assorted industrial wastes. And if information is poor and contentious concerning the average run of drugs, the situation with outlaw drugs is even more hopeless.

To complicate the situation even further, the decomposition of authority has become so advanced that the most honest and altruistic advice offered on drugs will be *disbelieved*, on principle, by large numbers of young people simply because it appears in the press or because it comes from somebody over thirty or because it issues from an established institution. This disbelief is by no means as irrational as might appear on the surface; on the contrary it reflects what may be taken as a healthy and much needed scepticism on the part of ordinary people to the authoritarianism of corporate bureaucrats and occult 'experts' who like to 'administer' human beings on the basis of their superior technological powers and alleged command over information – if the anarchic scepticism of the young forces this new priesthood of social engineers to become more open and responsive and human, this will be all to the good. The essence of the youthful critique of authority centres on hypocrisy. The essential hypocrisy of the adult world in dealing with drugs is the juxtaposition of unctuous paternalistic concern and savage moral outrage on the one hand with a dissolute degree of self-indulgence in alcohol, tobacco, pep pills, aspirins, tranquillizers, coffee, television and all other such opiates of the drug culture. It is hardly surprising then that when the Addiction Research Foundation conducted a study of drug use in Toronto schools they found that "the attitudes of parents toward tobacco, alcohol, and tranquillizers was found to relate directly to the way students approached drugs. For instance, more users than expected indicated that the parent or parents used both tobacco and alcohol. Those students who said they would not use drugs generally had parents who used neither alcohol nor tobacco."[22] Nor is it any more surprising that the same study found that while seven per cent had used marijuana, seven per cent speed, six per cent glue, and only three per cent LSD, at least forty-six per cent had used alcohol and thirty-eight per cent tobacco, demonstrating that tobacco and alcohol were the most used drugs, at "every grade level and for both sexes".[23] Those who would argue that bringing alcohol and cigarettes into a discussion of drug abuse is a diversion miss the real point. If education is going to be of any use, then part of the education process will have to involve a change in the adult world.

When a beer baron whose advertisements fill the media rises in the Senate to suggest a law that would make it a criminal offence to broadcast, print, or even – as was blandly suggested by one Senator – to *say* anything that is not wholly unfavorable concerning LSD, there are not many intelligent young people who will not immediately detect the conscious or unconscious hypocrisy of such an action. When a leading pharmaceutical firm that has grown fat on the sales of pep pills to adult pillheads publishes a booklet suggesting teachers turn in their kids to the cops if they catch them with pot,[24] what chance is there for such 'education' to be acceptable?

Alcohol has been almost as important a factor in Canadian history as wheat. Not only was the whiskey bottle a weapon against the Indians, not only was Sir John A. Macdonald a notorious, though lovable drunkard, but Confederation itself was virtually set afloat on an alcoholic sea. As the historian P. B. Waite describes the Charlottetown Conference of 1864:

Nothing was spared then, or later, to do whatever could be done with good food and good wine to make Islanders like Canadians, or Nova Scotians appreciate New Brunswickers . . . In those opulent days, before prohibition and taxes, no one was disposed to stint either in the provision or in the consumption of wine and spirits . . . The Canadian Cabinet never hesitated when it came to a few thousand dollars for entertainment; enough members of it were convinced that splendid intoxication was splendour sufficient for ordinary mortals, newly acquainted, and engaged in portentous public business. At four o'clock lunch began on the *Queen Victoria* . . . everyone was in good spirits; champagne corks punctuated the talk which soon waxed merrily . . . in the warmth of eloquence and champagne, the ice melted completely. The occasion took hold of everyone; so much so that the banns of union were read, and when no one demurred the British North American provinces were declared affianced and so it was proclaimed.

This luncheon on the *Queen Victoria* in Charlottetown harbour was, in a significant sense, the beginning of Confederation.[25]

Whether Confederation would have occurred in the cold light of sobriety remains a question mark, but it was neither the first nor the last time that a seduction was effected with the aid of liquor.

The previous paragraph was a test. The reaction of most readers was no doubt an indulgent chuckle. I would go further and suggest that the reaction even of those most vociferously concerned with the 'drug menace' would probably be an indulgent chuckle. *And this attitude is precisely the hypocrisy that makes any self-righteous education campaign doomed from the start.* The point is not, of course, that we should impose prohibition or go about smashing up pubs with axes like Carrie Nation a few generations ago. But if the moderate use of alcohol need not be a bad thing, then those who wish to 'educate' young people against drug abuse had better start considering the concept that the moderate use of marijuana need not in itself be a bad thing or that an LSD experience need not mark out an individual as a moral freak and a criminal. Immoderate use of alcohol can be very bad both for the individual and for society as a whole. So too immoderate use of pot could be very bad. It is essential for everybody's well-being that alcohol or marijuana or any other chemical that alters consciousness be recognized as a potential waster of human life.

Only if the would-be teachers of the young come before their audience in complete honesty will the audience really *listen.* Only if they have the courage to say: "Look kids, we all have problems. You have them, we have them. Some of you smoke pot, or drop acid, or sniff glue, or chew Morning Glory seeds, or squirt orange juice into your veins, or eat nutmeg, and maybe some of you have even started shooting heroin. We drink Scotch and beer by the gallon, chain smoke cigarettes, work like hell at jobs we hate, buy useless merchandise until our houses are stuffed, and sit stupid in front of the television every night of our lives. But these aren't our *real* problems. Your pot and our booze are escapes. But they *can* become the main problem if we let them – you can end up as wasted and dying speed freaks or as stuporous, languid potheads; we can end up as decaying alcoholics or cancerous smokers. Why don't we get together instead? *You* tell *us* what *you* think and we'll listen and then tell you what *we* think. Like why you hate us, and why we're afraid of you. And if we bring it all up, vomit it up right in the open, then maybe we'll both get rid of all that stuff that's twisting up our insides, and then maybe we'll both learn something, not only about each other, but about ourselves."

Only if . . . But don't hold your breath until it happens.

A Toronto student told a researcher, "I don't think adults realize that we know more than they think. If you come out with something about drugs or alcohol or anything at home they look at you. That's half the trouble; they push it away and say it's dirty so the kids turn around and find out from their friends or try it themselves."[26] In the same study it was found that one quarter of students surveyed referred to their friends as their most reliable source of information on drugs. The more unobtainable the drug concerned, the more important the peer group is as a source of information. Only 8.5 per cent thought that schools had contributed to their knowledge. Yet the overwhelming majority, 84 per cent, thought that drug education should begin in grade nine or earlier.[27]

Three dimensions of the education problem can be glimpsed by the following items. The Vancouver School Board has been operating a drug education program since 1966, which attempts to operate on a relatively low-key basis so that the drug problem will not appear to be a crisis situation but can be discussed calmly and matter-of-factly.[28] The Montreal Protestant School Board has stated its belief that "only factual information well presented, and not conjecture based on an emotional appeal, will have an influence on our young people today."[29] Asked what kind of information students would accept on drugs, a consultant to the North York Board of Education in Toronto said "it isn't information students require, it's example."[30] All these points are valid, but none is enough in itself, and fitting together all the requirements of a good educational program is a delicate balancing act. As the Executive Director of the Addiction Research Foundation has stated:

Today's young people do not believe dogmatic statements — especially when it is so easy to find contradictory statements that are equally dogmatic. The 'scare' technique — warning against dire consequences of drug use — is not very persuasive, since many young people are likely to know persons who have used these drugs without apparent adverse effects. Discussion is inevitable; and what is important is to ensure that discussion will be well-informed and will make sense in relation to youthful needs and aspirations. As one researcher has commented, many young people do not use drugs and perhaps never will; but they respect many of the views expressed by, or associated with, the drug users.[31]

Another official of the same organization came to the core of the problem when he advised teachers to quit laying down the law to young people and give them the opportunity of making up their own minds. He defined education as the "process of developing a capacity within people to make their own decisions". But he added that much of the teaching on drug abuse "seeks to deprive young people of the right to make their own decisions."[32]

We are a long way from a genuine two-way educational system, liberated from the ossified and irrelevant authority structure of the past, in which both teachers and students interact in a creative dialectic. But at least there is light at the end of *this* tunnel. In the other direction there lies only repression and intolerance, and inevitable failure.

'You are old, father William, 'the young man said,
'And your hair has become very white;
And yet you incessantly stand on your head —
Do you think, at your age, it is right?'

'In my youth,' father William replied to his son,
'I feared it might damage the brain;
But, now that I'm perfectly sure I have none,
Why, I do it again and again.'[33]

Footnotes

[1]House of Commons, *Debates* (Oct. 17, 1968), p. 1464.

[2]Friedrich Nietzsche, *Beyond Good and Evil*, translated by Marianne Cowan. (Chicago, Henry Regnery Co., 1955) p. 85.

[3]R. v. McNicol (1968) 1 D.L.R. (3rd). 328. (Monnin, J. A.)

[4]R. v. Adelman (1968) 3 C.C.C., 311.63 W.W.R., 294.

[5]R. v. Hinch and Salanski (1967), 62 W.W.R. 205.

[6]*Criminal Law Quarterly*, vol. 11, no. 2 (Feb., 1969), p. 120.

[7]"West Hill girl, 18, told out of Yorkville," *Globe and Mail* (Nov. 11, 1967).

[8]"Judge slams advocates of legal pot," *Ottawa Citizen* (Oct. 1, 1968).

[9]Leader in *The Daily Telegraph* (July 17, 1967).

[10]"Less Stringent Marijuana laws are sought," *Ottawa Citizen* (Nov. 20, 1968).

[11]"Inquest rules smoking by intoxicated persons caused 3-death blaze," *Globe and Mail* (May 2, 1967).

[12]Senate of Canada, *Debates* (Nov. 1, 1967), p. 340.

[13]Robert de Ropp, *Drugs and the Mind* (New York, Grove Press, 1957), pp. 126-27.

[14]Bill Davidson, "The Hidden Evils of LSD," *Saturday Evening Post* (Aug. 12, 1967), p. 20.

[15]*British Medical Journal*, vol. 4 (1968), p. 339.

[16]"Marijuana caused man to drill hole in head, U.K. psychiatrist says," *Globe and Mail* (Aug. 5, 1967).

[17]Bob Cohen, "Chromosome damage in spacemen feared," *Ottawa Citizen* (Jan. 3, 1969).

[18]"No prosecution in LSD hoax, state decides," *Globe and Mail* (Jan. 31, 1968).

[19]"Lawless 'beat' generation must be controlled says RCMP Commissioner," *Ottawa Citizen* (Feb. 21, 1968).

[20]"Draft a health hazard," *Ottawa Citizen* (March 6, 1968).

[21]Rudy Platiel, "Some Questions," *Globe and Mail* (Jan. 23, 1969).

198 / *Drugs and the Law*

22Addiction Research Foundation, *A Preliminary Report on the Attitude and Behaviour of Toronto Students in Relation to Drugs* (Toronto, Jan., 1969), pp. 5-6.

23*Ibid.*, p. 2. My own impression — and it is no more than an impression — is that the use of outlawed drugs may be more widespread in the high schools than these figures indicate.

24"The Indecent Society," *The New Republic*, vol. 156, no. 19 (May 13, 1967), p. 5.

25P. B. Waite, *The Life and Times of Confederation, 1864-1867* (Toronto, University of Toronto Press, 1962), pp. 77-78.

26Addiction Research Foundation, *Preliminary Report, op. cit.*, p. 7.

27*Ibid.*, pp. 6-7

28John Clarke, "The educational approach to the growing drug problems in high schools," *Globe and Mail* (Feb. 1, 1969).

29Quoted in The Royal Bank of Canada, *Monthly Letter*, vol. 45, no. 9, p. 4.

30Joan Hollobon, "Sentences given for marijuana called ridiculous by judge," *Globe and Mail* (Feb. 22, 1969).

31H. D. Archibald, "Perspective on Marihuana," *Addictions*, vol. 15, no. 2 (Summer, 1968), pp. 4-5.

32"Don't lay down law about drugs, alcohol, teachers are advised," *Globe and Mail* (March 20, 1968). The official was Robert Robinson, director of education for the Foundation.

33Lewis Carroll, *Alice's Adventures in Wonderland*, in *The Works of Lewis Carroll* (London, Paul Hamlyn, 1965), p. 52.

Crimes Without Victims

Throughout this book we have been continually coming up against an apparent paradox: laws are being broken, crimes are being committed; but there are no victims who complain to the police. We generally think of crimes as some sort of aggression against an individual, as a wilful violation of a human being's person or property. When someone is murdered and the accused is standing trial, a certain amount of sympathy may be generated for the murderer as well as for the victim, if unfortunate circumstances are disclosed, but such sympathy generally stops short of condoning the act itself, for scarcely anyone ultimately questions the principle that murder itself is wrong. And this is equally true of most crimes that go on day after day in our society.

How then are we to react to the recent words of a County Judge in Whitby, Ontario, in apologizing to a man and wife convicted of possessing morphine.

Apparently I must do something which offends against every legal
instinct I know. Parliament has seen fit to make this an offence. . . . I find
it hard to find any legal principle for what I must do. . . . In cases such
as rape and assault, I can feel I am acting for the protection of society.
It is difficult for me to find where your actions have hurt anyone but
yourself. It is impossible for me to believe that any sentence I impose
today will deter others from committing like offences.[1]

What this uncommonly fair-minded judge was grappling with in his mind was a very old problem in the life of democratic countries: the conflict between our oft-expressed theory of a free and liberal social order, and the reality of a pervasive regulation of morality by the state. It is curious that in some of the more backward and reactionary autocracies in the world the tyrannized subjects have perhaps more personal freedom with regard to such matters as drinking, gambling, copulating, or otherwise choosing their own favorite path to Hell, than does the average citizen of a democracy – just so long, of course, that politics is avoided. Despite our pride in our political freedoms, it is astonishing to contemplate the list of prohibited personal actions that burden down our laws, and much of it without comment, much less complaint on the part of average citizens. Indeed, when the then Justice Minister, Pierre Elliott Trudeau, made his famous statement that "the state has no business in the bedrooms of the nation," it was as if a magic spell had been broken.

But the idea that in a democracy it is one of the prerogatives of the majority to regulate moral conduct and to punish any deviations from the norm is by no means dead; indeed it seems so deep-rooted in our society that when it has been removed from one area it tends to spring up again in a newer and more virulent form elsewhere. Thus at the very moment when the regulation and enforcement of a repressive sexual morality seems to be under attack and weakening, there is a rising clamor for more and more potent laws against any unapproved use of drugs.

We must face up to the fact that the Morality Squad mentality answers a fundamental need in democratic society, the need to raise up the image of the People-at-large, even at the expense of the individuals who make up the People. When Alexis de Tocqueville wrote his classic study of the infant American democracy of the early nineteenth century,[2] he warned his European audience that America was both the freest and at the same time the most despotic nation on earth. This paradox arose, suggested Tocqueville, because each democratic citizen believes that since he chooses his own government he is by definition free – yet on the other hand this same government acts as the oppressive instrument of the majority by minutely regulating the social and private lives of individuals, in the interests of 'equality', so that eventually all local and individual differences are eradicated. As in so much else of what he wrote, Tocqueville here cut directly to the heart of the matter. Parliament, free elections, a free press, are all very valuable, but when the voluntary and involuntary pressures toward social conformity are overwhelming, how free a people are we in reality?

What seems to have deeply offended the Whitby judge quoted

earlier was the way in which a moral judgment about private behavior ("drug addiction is a Bad Thing") has been written into a
body of law that purports to be the safeguard of individual liberty.
The two persons charged in the case had, of course, harmed nobody
other than themselves. But it is precisely here that the allegedly
liberal basis of our legal system begins to look a trifle threadbare.
If people are supposed to be free to live their own lives so long as
they do not interfere with the lives of others, one might assume that
this would imply the freedom to act in ways not approved by the
majority. This has, however, never really been a leading principle
of our society, outside of abstract philosophizing and patriotic
rhetoric. More to the point is the imaginary case described by British
humorist A. P. Herbert of the man who, to win a wager, jumped fully
clothed into the Thames, only to be arrested on the suspicion of
having done something or other contrary to law. In the considered
opinion of "Lord Justice Frog"

... the appellant made the general answer that this was a free country
and a man can do what he likes if he does nobody any harm ... it would
be idle to deny that a man capable of that remark would be capable of
the grossest forms of licence and disorder. It cannot be too clearly
understood that this is *not* a free country, and it will be an evil day for
the legal profession when it is. The citizens of London must realize that
there is almost nothing they are allowed to do. *Prima facie* all actions are
illegal, if not by Act of Parliament, by Order in Council; and if not by
Order in Council, by Departmental or Police Regulations, or By-laws. They
may not eat where they like, drink where they like, walk where they like,
drive where they like, sing where they like, or sleep where they like. And
least of all may they do unusual actions 'for fun'. People must not do
things for fun. We are not here for fun. There is no reference to fun in any
Act of Parliament. And if anything is said in this Court to encourage a
belief that Englishmen are entitled to jump off bridges for their own
amusement the next thing to go will be the Constitution. For these reasons,
therefore, I have to come to the conclusion that this appeal must fail.
It is not for me to say what offence the appellant has committed, but
I am satisfied that he has committed *some* offence, for which he has
been most properly punished.

   Mudd, J., said that in his opinion the appellant had done his trousers
no good and the offence was damage to property....

   The appeal was dismissed.[3]

   More seriously, offences regarding drugs fall into a general
category of acts that might be called *crimes without victims*, that

is, 'crimes' in which there are no injured or complaining parties. Other activities that fall into the same category are abortion, prostitution, gambling, and until recently, homosexuality. What is common to all these activities is a situation in which one person obtains from another, in an exchange, a commodity or service that is officially considered to be immoral. A characteristic of all such crimes without victims is the unenforceability of the laws. This derives directly from the lack of a complaint and the obvious difficulty in obtaining evidence.[4]

There are a vast number of acts commonly undertaken by private citizens that might be interpreted as counter to the generally accepted moral code. All such acts, however, are not in fact prohibited by law. Only a few are selectively made the subject of legislation. One might wonder by what process society moves from a general moral value to a specific act of enforcement. One sociologist, Howard Becker, has suggested that at certain times, certain persons have undertaken the role of 'moral entrepreneurs', those who have made it their business to ensure that specific legal rules are deduced and enacted. The motives of such moral entrepreneurs have usually been based on the desire to bring society into line with the Protestant ethic of self-control, which views pleasure as moral only when it serves as a reward for work. Such a desire has often been expressed in terms of reform and humanitarianism, and has just as often been accepted as a valid exercise in do-goodism. Becker cites the role of the U.S. Narcotics Bureau in bringing into being a specific prohibition of marijuana in the late 1930s and notes how the Bureau manipulated public opinion through the press by the circulation of atrocity stories designed to spread the idea that marijuana was extremely dangerous and immoral. The resulting moral indignation of voters was then used as an instrument for the passage of strong anti-marijuana laws through the U.S. Congress and state legislatures. The entire campaign was waged amid an aura of a great moral reform.[5] Of course, the Narcotics Bureau, whose appropriations had been steadily declining, stood to gain significantly from the grant of a wide new area of jurisdiction, and from the addition of a new justification for its continued bureaucratic existence. Such a mixture of motives is common in such cases.

Joseph Gusfield, in a study of the long-lived American temperance movement, has suggested that pluralistic democracies are faced with the special problem of competing 'life styles' among the various co-existing subcultures within society. Instead of the pure class conflict often seen in European countries between the bourgeoisie and the workers, North American society is often characterized by a struggle among competing status groups, each attempting to assert the supremacy of its own way of life, and, by implication, the illegitimacy of all other ways of life. Since economic issues are often secondary, the struggle then becomes a clash between the visible symbols of competing life styles. Gusfield thus relates the struggle for Prohibition in the United States with the desire of the older rural society to maintain ascendancy over the newer, more permissive urban culture of the twentieth century, by focussing on alcohol as the symbol of urban life.

As his own claim to social respect and honour are diminished, the sober, abstaining citizen seeks for public acts through which he may reaffirm the dominance and prestige of his style of life. Converting the sinner to virtue is one way; law is another. Even if the law is not enforced or enforceable, the symbolic import of its passage is important to the reformer. It settles the controversies between those who represent clashing cultures. The public support of one conception of morality at the expense of another enhances the prestige and self-esteem of the victors and degrades the culture of the losers.[6]

The aim of such legislation is always proclaimed to be the elimination of the behavior in question, but this goal is never reached. The reason for such continuing failure is not hard to find: all the law can really do is to regulate the conditions under which prohibited exchanges take place, since the *demand* for the illegal goods or services is not eliminated by the mere passage of a law. It is an easily verifiable observation that drug addicts get their drugs, law or no law. Instead of getting a certified dose at a reasonable price from an accredited medical doctor within the context of medical therapy, the addict instead buys a commodity of unknown quality and dubious content from a street seller for a viciously prohibitive price. These conditions, of course, do not discourage the addict, since his demand for opiates is inelastic, that is, it exists without regard to the conditions of supply. But the form of regulation adopted under our laws has the effect of defining the problem of drug addiction in ways that have little to do with the problem itself. The addict becomes, by decree, a criminal. An addict subculture springs up, which contributes strongly to the continuation and reinforcement of addiction, even though such a subculture is more a product of the law than of the phenomenon of addiction itself.

Because there is no evidence from complaining victims, the police are forced to use extraordinary methods of investigation, such as the use of undercover agents and entrapment of suspects by police offers to buy drugs – methods that often raise questions both of civil liberties and of simple propriety. The police are in a most peculiar position altogether, since they cannot possibly be effective in combatting such crimes using normal police methods that suffice for the general run of robberies and muggings, while on the other hand they can never be wholly effective no matter how relentless their methods, since the *demand* for drugs, or for abortions, or for prostitution, or for gambling, is simply not eliminated by legislative fiat. We thus end up with the highly unsatisfactory situation of a disproportionate amount of police time and resources spent on combatting actions on the part of individuals which may harm themselves but generally speaking do not cause harm to others. Worse, the large establishment necessary to carry on such a hopeless law enforcement campaign becomes itself a vested interest, which to maintain its continued claims upon the public purse must annually assert that: (a) it is doing an effective job in eliminating the drug manace, but that: (b) a substantial menace nevertheless continues to exist, necessitating the enforcement agency's continued operation and perhaps even justifying its expansion. It is all slightly reminiscent of the role of the U.S. military in the alleged supression of the Viet Cong.

In their own defence the police often assert that they do not make the law, but only enforce it. Strictly speaking this is, of course, true. But on the other hand, the police, both RCMP and metropolitan police departments, are quick to add their voices to political debate against any proposed liberalization of the laws concerning drug abuse, and are just as quick to suggest tougher laws and more extensive police powers.[7] In this sense, the police are not acting as mere passive agents of parliament, because the voices of police spokesmen obviously carry considerable weight with legislators. The problem is that the police appear to believe in the validity of laws regulating moral conduct;[8] they thus tend to view the matter as essentially *how* the given laws are to be most effectively and efficiently enforced. But in so doing the police are in fact helping to perpetuate a considerable problem for themselves.

It has become apparent in recent years that a crisis of authority has grown up around the role of the police in Canadian society. It is a common observation that the public at large, and particularly young people, are losing respect for the police both as individuals and as symbols of legitimate authority. It is understandable that in this situation the police feel angry and beleaguered. It is also understandable that they should associate this breakdown of authority with a moral fault on the part of young people and conclude that the restoration of authority can be accomplished through external discipline and the exercise of coercive power to enforce a standard of behavior approved by the majority. Perhaps for the first time a significant section of middle-class society, teen-agers and students in particular, are evolving a life-style in sharp contrast to that style usually considered 'normal'. Drugs, especially marijuana, have a certain place in this life-style. The result is that a section of middle-class society is beginning to perceive the police, not as the defenders of their lives and property, but as coercive agents enforcing an unwanted personal morality on people who have already rejected it. The concept of treating drug addicts as criminals has been largely accepted for years since most narcotics users were working-class slum dwellers. When middle-class youth is arrested in relatively large numbers on narcotics charges, the inequity of crimes without victims becomes more widely perceived, and the authority of the police, the most visible symbol of this inequity, begins to crumble. Children have been brought up in our society to despise the secret police methods employed in 'totalitarian' countries, only to find that their own government condones such practices as planting undercover agents to win the confidence of unsuspecting youths in order to entrap them in illegal acts – when in fact such acts are often undertaken at the direct instigation of the agent. Is it any wonder then that under such circumstances there is a crisis of authority? That fear and hatred of the law has sprung up among at least one section of middle-class youth? That such fear and hatred is vented on the police?

The situation is in essence tragic. The police are being blamed for attempting to enforce laws that are basically unenforceable and authoritarian by nature. Yet the police are themselves rarely able to understand that it is the role they are expected to play as regulators of morality that causes the breakdown of their authority. The only solution they seem to perceive to this dilemma is the passage of tougher laws and the grant of more powers of enforcement. There is something sadly futile in the spectacle of youth committed to meaningful social change locked in an endless struggle with the police whom they begin to see as the enemy incarnate, while at the same time the police sometimes seem convinced that long hair and marijuana are at the root of moral decay in our civilization. The police end up by acting as the willing agents of those who project all their discontent and guilt onto 'long-haired', 'rebellious' youth; and at the same time youth plays along by focussing on the cop as the target of protest and abuse. The squalid scenes outside the Democratic Convention in Chicago in 1968 were the final culmination of this mentality: the protesters throwing out such wise slogans as Pig and the police replying with clubs and fists.

Yet this is surely a vicious circle. The police, after all, are neither the directors nor the beneficiaries of the North American political and economic system. They are not especially well paid, their working conditions are difficult, and their job does not even bring much prestige. They are hardly, then, a legitimate target for youthful protest. On the other hand, so long as the police are expected to act as the enforcers of morality in areas that are essentially personal in nature, they will inevitably be viewed as threats to the liberty of individuals.

Ultimately the point is that the police are not qualified to be the arbiters of private morality. To say this is not to disparage the police, any more than the statement that engineers are not qualified to teach music appreciation constitutes a criticism of their social value as engineers. By background, by training, by motivation, the police are simply not qualified to dictate what values private citizens ought to accept, if indeed anyone is so qualified. If this unenviable role were to be taken out of their hands, it could be the police themselves who would gain the most. For they could then concentrate on their essentially honorable role as the guardians of life, limb, and property – a role which, if exercized even-handedly, ought to inspire respect. This is not to suggest that the entire problem of police authority and respect would be thus solved since there are probably more fundamental reasons involved, but a diminution of their more unpopular functions would certainly help. And drugs would be a good place to start.

There is yet another, darker, side to the place of crimes without victims in contemporary society. There is a good deal of current agitation about the growing power of organized crime in this country. But amid all the alarms and exhortations there does not seem to have been very much hard thinking about what organized crime feeds on. In fact it is generally recognized that three pillars of organized criminal activity on this continent are gambling, prostitution, and narcotics. What in fact could be more made-to-measure for the enterprising crime syndicate than the existence of a widespread demand for prohibited goods and services, with laws and law enforcement acting exactly as a protective tariff, ensuring that exorbitant and highly profitable prices may be charged? In this sense, organized crime is simply acting in the same way as any legitimate business concern, by efficiently providing for the distribution of goods and services for which a demand exists – except that in this case the goods and services are declared to be illegitimate. Despite general pronouncements of moral intent, however, a widespread demand will continue to exist for such goods and services, since the demand is founded on private needs, in the face of which social approval or disapproval is simply irrelevant.

So long, for example, as there are women who want and need abortions, there will be those ready to provide the service. Women have abortions in Japan, where there is apparently no social disapproval. Women also have abortions in Canada, where there is considerable social disapproval, backed by the criminal sanction. The only real difference is in the quality of the services provided and the price attached. Since the Canadian abortionist is an illegal operator his methods are unsupervised and the threat of arrest constitutes a high overhead cost of his operations, which in turn means an extremely high price. Thus poor people, who can often least afford to provide for children, often find it difficult to pay for abortion, while the rich can easily absorb the cost.

Up to now it does not appear that organized crime has gone into the business of providing abortions. Perhaps if it had, the cost might have been lowered since a large-scale organization might conceivably rationalize the present chaotic distribution of such services. On the other hand, perhaps a monopoly situation might raise the price, while the present system of competition among many sellers may have kept the cost down. All in all an interesting problem for economists, but one that points up an essential aspect of the actual impact of all laws such as that against abortion: all that is really accomplished is a type of government regulation of the market.

And it is a type of regulation that, especially in the case of narcotics, as well as gambling and prostitution, paves the way for organized crime. At the moment the production and distribution of marijuana and LSD is essentially in the hands of the same people who buy the goods. It is safe to suggest that any significant tightening of the laws and of law enforcement would only make it more likely that organized crime would begin to move into the market, since it possesses entrepreneurial talents appropriate to a situation of high risk.

The obvious way to undercut any business is to steal its market; it is thus surprising that a business-oriented society like our own has not hit upon the obvious way to strike a blow at organized crime where it really hurts – in the pocketbook – by the simple expedient of rendering some of its major activities unprofitable. This can be done by allowing the controlled and supervised distribution of some hitherto prohibited goods and services, such as narcotics.

The public, and most certainly the police, could be expected to respond to such a suggestion in a predictable manner: it is unthinkable and immoral to legalize criminal activity. Here we really get to the root of the problem, for there is no more firmly planted fallacy than the belief that crime is, like disease, a phenomenon of nature. Crime is *not* like disease; crime is a man-made concept, defined by law. Legislatures create crime, strictly speaking, by declaring certain activities to be criminal. Yet the crime rate is spoken of as being on the increase in the same way that the progress of influenza epidemics is charted, without any apparent realization that the official authorities hold it within their power to decrease the crime rate by the simple expedient of repealing a number of laws. Now to be sure, there is excellent reason for the criminal sanction being applied to most current offences, but the category of crimes without victims represents a very different face altogether.[9]

The question should not be, "do you disapprove of drug abuse and therefore approve of tough laws against it?" There are in fact two separate questions involved here, and distinctions must be made. It can be argued, and has been argued earlier in this book, that our present method of dealing with illicit drug use may very well have made the problem much worse than it would otherwise have been. 'Legalizing' opiate use, to use the vulgarization usually applied to the method of placing the addict within a voluntary context of medical treatment, promises far more in terms of actually dealing with the problem. It is moreover a fallacy that 'legalizing' a commodity or service now prohibited under law in any way implies that social disapproval has been transformed into social approval. The point is that the law does not work, and brings in its wake a host of undesirable side-effects, and that there is no overwhelming reason why other, non-coercive measures could not be tried. To argue that the 'legalization' of, say, marijuana use means that society will thus be giving its approval to the practice is about as sensible as arguing that anything not specifically prohibited by law must therefore be socially approved. It is not a criminal offence to be an alcoholic – does this mean that society wishes to encourage people to become alcoholics? Obviously not, and removing all legal penalties on marijuana would not imply social 'approval' of marijuana misuse; it would merely imply a realistic recognition of the limits of the criminal sanction in dealing with this particular problem, and perhaps a recognition of the degree to which private behavior can in fact be treated simply as private behavior, without the necessity of passing moral judgments upon it.

Unfortunately, in the real world, it is not as simple as mere abstract logic would suggest. It is all very well for legislators to say, "well, we have a drug problem: why don't we try making the whole business illegal and see how that works out." In fact, when laws were first passed against opium in this country, such an experimental attitude was uppermost in many minds, just as today the government turns over liberalization and tougher laws in its mind as possible alternative solutions to the hallucinogenic drug issue. The problem is, however, that the idea of passing a law, watching the results, and, if they are not encouraging, scrapping the prohibition approach after a few years of testing, turns out to be extremely difficult in practice. This is because the public normally considers anything that is illegal to be intrinsically immoral. Thus the illegality of opiates has resulted in an aura of evil and criminality surrounding drug addiction. Similarly the passage of laws against LSD has made legitimate medical and psychological research employing LSD difficult as well as suspect in the eyes of the public. The illegality of marijuana has made a public discussion of the drug painfully difficult – many people simply refuse to even listen to arguments for the legalization of marijuana use since they feel that such arguments constitute a plea for the unleashing of crime and lawlessness, and they assume that any liberalization is the equivalent of surrendering society to the ravages of disease. In fact, there is a most depressing tendency for any debate on such matters to degenerate to the level of "are you or are you not against sin?"

What happens then is that experiments in drug prohibition tend to be self-perpetuating, and we end up with a tangled knot of law, moralism, and misconceptions that is very difficult to untangle Unfortunately, the tendency always seems to be toward more, rather than fewer, laws. The most common attitude when faced with any type of behavior that is unfamiliar or bizarre is summed up in the familiar expression "there ought to be a law". But like bureaucratic institutions, old laws rarely die or even fade away. Instead they linger on indefinitely, guarded by those organizations with a vested interest in maintaining them, by the public conception that anything illegal must be immoral, and by sheer deadly inertia. Perhaps we need some clear-headed Alexander to simply slice this Gordian knot through at one stroke. But at least our legislators ought to be extremely cautious and circumspect in considering new laws to ban new drugs.[10]

Up to this point we have been proceeding on the assumption that crimes without victims are in fact both a violation of individual liberty and an illegitimate, or at least inadvisable, use of the criminal sanction. The reader may well object that this assumption has not been proved and that perhaps there are compelling reasons for society to enforce an approved set of morals in the realm of private behavior. We have postponed consideration of this question until the end because it raises some fundamental points, many of which go beyond the scope of this work. Some points, however, we will try to deal with.

The first, and no doubt the greatest, modern attempt to define the theoretical distinction between law and morality, was made by John Stuart Mill, who was deeply concerned by the social conformity and tyranny of public opinion that he saw around him in Victorian England. Fearful of a trend toward the legislation of morals, Mill put forward the following proposition.

The object . . . is to assert one very simple principle, as entitled to
govern absolutely the dealings of society with the individual in the way
of compulsion and control, whether the means used be physical force
in the form of legal penalties, or the moral coercion of public opinion.
That principle is, that the sole end for which mankind are warranted,

*individually or collectively, in interfering with the liberty of action of
any of their number, is self-protection. That the only purpose for which
power can be rightfully exercised over any member of a civilised
community, against his will, is to prevent harm to others.* His own good,
either physical or moral, is not a sufficient warrant. He cannot
rightfully be compelled to do or forbear because it would be better for
him to do so, because it will make him happier, because, in the opinion
of others, to do so would be wise, or even right. These are good reasons
for remonstrating with him, or reasoning with him, or persuading him,
or entreating him, but not for compelling him, or visiting him with any
evil in case he can do otherwise. To justify that, the conduct from which it
is desired to deter him must be calculated to produce evil to some one else.
The only part of the conduct of any one, for which he is amenable to
society, is that which concerns others. In the part which merely concerns
himself, his independence is, of right, absolute. Over himself, over his
own body and mind, the individual is sovereign.[11] (Italics mine)

Mill was clearly stating an abstract, rationalistic theory of what the
limits of the law *ought to be*. Critics of Mill have sometimes pointed
out that the law does not now, and never has, recognized the limits
laid down by Mill. This is obviously true, but irrelevant, since Mill
was not describing, but prescribing. At the heart of Mill's theory lay
the notion that morality could not be frozen by act of parliament,
that the way must be open for, as he put it, "experiments in living".
We cannot ever be absolutely certain about the ultimate validity of
any moral proposition any more than we can be certain about the
ultimate validity of any scientific hypothesis. There must be freedom
of inquiry; the only limit is that no one else be harmed. On this fundamental proposition of nineteenth-century liberalism much of the
case against crimes without victims still rests.

It is only recently that the debate generated by Mill in the latter
part of the last century has been resumed, and it is perhaps fitting
that it has taken place among two of Mill's countrymen. Lord Devlin,
a judge of the Queen's Bench and more recently a Lord of Appeal,
has severely criticized Mill's views and strongly upheld the right,
and the obligation of society to enforce morality by means of the
criminal sanction. Lord Devlin denies that private morality can be
equated to private religious belief as being no concern of the State.
A society can practise religious tolerance and survive, but the same
is not true of moral permissiveness. For to Lord Devlin, positive
morality is the cement that holds any society together. To preserve

itself, society must therefore enforce its morality through the coercive sanctions of the law.

Society is entitled by means of its laws to protect itself from dangers, whether from within or without ... An established morality is as necessary as good government to the welfare of society. Societies disintegrate from within more frequently than they are broken up by external pressures. There is disintegration when no common morality is observed and history shows that the loosening of moral bonds is often the first stage of disintegration, so that society is justified in taking the same steps to preserve its moral code as it does to preserve its government and other essential institutions. The suppression of vice is as much the law's business as the suppression of subversive activities; it is no more possible to define a sphere of private morality than it is to define one of private subversive activity ... There are no theoretical limits to the power of the State to legislate against treason and sedition, and likewise I think there can be no theoretical limits to legislation against morality.[12]

Actually, Lord Devlin is not a totalitarian, and he does set a practical limit to State intervention: enforcement should only take place when the behavior in question is not merely distasteful but actually repugnant to society in general. The determination of the degree of such repugnance is left to a jury of average citizens, to the "reasonable man," who, Lord Devlin is quick to point out, is by no means synonymous with the rational man. Lord Devlin thus reduces the problem from a question of *values* to a question of *facts*. The lawyer is concerned not with law as it *ought* to be, but with law as it *is*. Similarly, the legislator is not concerned with morality as it ought to be, but as it is in fact. Those who serve the law "do not look up too often to the heights of what ought to be lest they lose sight of the ground on which they stand and which it is their duty to defend – the law as it is, morality as it is, freedom as it is – none of them perfect but the things their society has got and must not let go."[13] In short, if any behavior – in our case presumably drug addiction or illicit drug use – rouses feelings of "intolerance, indignation, and disgust"[14] on the part of the average citizen, then the State has a duty to legislate against such behavior.

H. L. A. Hart, Professor of Jurisprudence at Oxford, replied to Lord Devlin's attack on Mill by denying that there is a necessary connection between the general social interest in a shared morality and the enforcement of any particular moral principle. Morality in fact changes, but society continues. Hart suggests that Lord Devlin, and others like him, make the mistake of assuming that morality is a "seamless web" that must be maintained without amendment. Even the great conservative philosopher Edmund Burke would not have accepted such a view, according to Hart: "To use coercion to maintain the moral *status quo* at any point in a society's history would be artificially to arrest the process which gives social institutions their value."[15] Worse, Lord Devlin's designation of "the ordinary citizen, and more specifically, of the feelings of "intolerance, indignation, and disgust" on the part of the ordinary citizen, as the indication of whether private acts should be punished, represents a kind of moral populism that if given free reign, would no doubt destroy all the liberties which the individual presently enjoys. We referred earlier in this chapter to Tocqueville's characterization of American democracy as both free and despotic. Clearly Lord Devlin stands with those forces that favor the People-at-large as against the individual.

Hart basically upholds the position of John Stuart Mill, but with one exception – unlike Mill, Hart admits that *paternalism*, the notion that the State can protect the individual against himself, is a valid basis for legislation. Thus he specifically criticizes Mill's view that any restrictions on the sale of drugs are an interference with the liberty of the purchaser, and suggests that paternalism toward the purchaser is the explanation for restrictions on narcotics rather than the desire of society to punish the seller for his immorality. It might seem then that both Hart and Devlin are in agreement on the validity of anti-drug legislation. It must be remembered, however, that Hart was writing about *English* law and that the British system of dealing with opiates has been based on a distinction between legal medically-prescribed use and illegal non-prescribed use.

I think, along with Hart, that it is no longer possible to maintain that any restriction on the sale of drugs is an unjustifiable violation of the purchaser's liberty. If heroin and other opiates were sold freely across the counter of the local drug store there would quite probably be a dreadful increase in drug addiction. Indeed this is precisely what happened in the nineteenth century and there can be no doubt that the outlawing of nonmedical opiate distribution has led to a decrease in the overall addiction rate. We have gone too far down the road of paternalism in all aspects of life – welfare, health services, education – to tolerate the unrestricted and unregulated distribution of a commodity that plays a part in the creation of a major health problem, that the State itself is usually obligated to deal with in terms of treatment and prevention. It does not seem logical to state, on the one hand that individuals have a right to state-supported health services and on the other that they have a right to freely experiment with substances that may drastically impair their health. The LSD users may speak of their right to experiment with their own minds, but when these experiments go wrong, as they sometimes do, it is the State that must often look after them – and in some cases this may turn out to be a very long-term proposition. The community, and the taxpayers, have rights as well.

As Hart points out, Mill wrote *On Liberty* in the era of Victorian liberal optimism, when a good deal more faith was vested in human reason and in the durability of human values than we are now able to accept. There as been

... a general decline in the belief that individuals know their own interests best, and ... an increased awareness of a great range of factors which diminish the significance to be attached to an apparently free choice or to consent. Choices may be made or consent given without adequate reflection or appreciation of the consequences; or in pursuit of merely transitory desires; or in various predicaments when the judgment is likely to be clouded; or under inner psychological compulsion; or under pressure by others of a kind too subtle to be susceptible of proof in a law court. Underlying Mill's extreme fear of paternalism there perhaps is a conception of what a normal human being is like which now seems not to correspond to the facts. Mill, in fact, endows him with too much of the psychology of a middle-aged man whose desires are relatively fixed, not liable to be artificially stimulated by external influences; who knows what he wants and what gives him satisfaction or happiness; and who pursues these things when he can.[16]

Hart's point is, I think, well taken. It should be recognized, however, that Hart is not suggesting that the State may legislate against drug use on the grounds that drug use is *immoral*, but rather that the State may be able to protect an individual against his own weakness or lack of knowledge. But if we cannot argue that the State has no right to interfere with the sale of drugs, we certainly can raise some serious questions as to the *efficacy* of the present method of legal regulation here in Canada.

It is a strange type of paternalism that makes sick people hunted criminals. It is a strange type of paternalism that declares that legislators, judges, and policemen should treat drug problems, but not medical doctors, psychologists, and sociologists. And it is a strange type of paternalism that says that the individual can best be protected from himself by kicking the hell out of him. While our ideas of the rationality of the individual may have changed since Mill's time, so too our idea of how the individual may be helped has changed. For all the reasons already outlined in this book it should be clear that the use of stern punishment as the major ingredient of drug therapy has proved to be a general disaster.

If paternalism is indeed the rationale of our approach to drug problems then it is a grievously mistaken notion of paternalism. But it is hard to escape the feeling that Lord Devlin may have a point when he speaks of the feelings of "intolerance, indignation and disgust" on the part of the average citizen as the real basis for laws such as those against drug use. Lord Devlin, of course, supports this as both just and useful. But even if one finds it difficult to positively support such emotions, it may be that they are *in fact* the real basis for much of our treatment of drug problems. If we were really interested in treating the problem in a rational manner it is doubtful that punishment and vengeance would occupy the centre of the stage.

It has already been maintained at some length that in the case of crimes without victims the law does not eliminate the proscribed behavior but merely regulates it, often in unintended ways. When one considers the dismal prospect of the opiate addict who is arrested, sent to prison or even to compulsory treatment centres, 'cured', and then arrested again and again in dreary succession, without any real attempt to come to grips with the underlying causes of addiction; when one considers the large number of young people given prison sentences and criminal records for marijuana use, without any real attempt to understand why they feel compelled to experiment with drugs; when one considers the sheer bloodthirstiness of so many legislators, judges, magistrates, policemen and opinion-makers when faced with the question of what to do with drug users; when one considers the fear, reluctance, and outright aversion that hospitals and private doctors sometimes have toward treating drug problems; when one considers the utter hopelessness of all attempts to eliminate private drug use by means of police coercion, and the virtual certainty that only an unlucky few will be punished for the sins of the many; when one considers all these factors, it is very difficult indeed to believe that our present approach is founded upon rational principles, either paternalistic or preventive.

However unsettling the prospect, it may be much more to the point to view the entire phenomenon as an elaborate social ceremony, in which the regular solid citizen continually re-establishes his identity and continually re-affirms his normality and membership in the society through the ritual isolation, purging, and expulsion of the abnormal, deviant individual. The myths that are built up around the 'dope-fiend', now reincarnated in the symbolic figure of the anarchic, long-haired, unclean, rebellious youth, become an amalgam of all that the God-fearing, tax-paying citizen most deeply fears: disorder, defiance, and above all else the liberation of pleasure from work. It is one of the most fundamental tenets of the Protestant ethic and thus of our business civilization that pleasure is only legitimate when given in reward for work. Yet alcohol use (pleasure in a bottle) has become intrinsic to our social life. The same guilt feelings that find uneasy expression in jokes about drunkenness also fix upon the half-mythical figure of the dope-fiend as their scapegoat. Such feelings become especially insistent with regard to youth who have not yet 'earned' their right to pleasure. Just as the white man has needed the Negro and the Indian on the bottom of the social order as a visible sign of his own superiority and his own intrinsic worth, so too the ordinary citizen *needs* the dope-fiend, upon whom he can project guilt feelings about his own weaknesses and inability to live up to the impossible demands of a repressive, work-dominated morality. The law ensures that such scapegoats are kept in constant supply, as it provides neither for the resolution of the social and economic problems that give rise to drug use, nor for the medical setting in which drug problems may be treated. Worse, by its policy of punishment and retribution, it ensures the further alienation of the drug user, and his consequent immersion within a drug subculture that sustains and reinforces his dependence on drug use. Rationalists who think that black magic is restricted to so-called 'primitive' societies would do well to ponder the social creation of the dope-fiend as scapegoat, and the kind of ethos that encourages a high police official to inform an assembly of school children that the "only cured addict is a dead addict".[17]

If there is any ray of light in this dark situation it is that the technological basis of the repressive work ethic upon which this scapegoat ceremony rests is itself changing. With automation, the necessity for a society to regiment its members as instruments of industrial production becomes less and less justifiable, for there are fewer and fewer jobs into which they may be fitted. It has become a commonplace that from a society of producers we are being transformed into a society of consumers, and consumers with the prospect of a great deal of leisure as well. It is at least possible that in this future in which pleasure is separated from work we may at last be able to come to terms with the necessary social and psychological function of mind-altering drugs, whether alcoholic, psychedelic, or whatever.

But if the social environment changes, it does not change at an even pace. It is precisely this unevenness that accounts for the strains we are experiencing today. The young, who see the world with fewer preconceptions and fewer inhibitions, are already adapting themselves for a future in which neither Horatio Alger nor John Calvin will have much place. To those who hold fast to the standard of hard work, success, and keeping your mouth shut, the behavior of the young seems to embody some undefined but menacing challenge.

The French anthropologist Lévi-Strauss was recently asked if anthropology were not a dying science due to the relentless 'modernization' of preliterate cultures all over the world. Lévi-Strauss replied that:

It is quite possible that there is a regulating principle in mankind, what I would call a principle of diversity, which would make it compulsory for differences to appear within this world-wide society to compensate to some extent for its uniformity. Perhaps this will take place in completely unforeseen ways. It is not at all impossible, for instance, that the kind of gap which we are now witnessing between the generations is a transposition in time of what was taking place earlier on in space. The tremendous development of communications makes it much easier for the younger generation to build up a culture of its own different from the culture of the previous generation. So in that case we will still have diversity to work with.[18]

There was once a time in Europe when questions of religious belief tore whole societies apart. Religious warfare was finally avoided by the secularization of society, and religious tolerance. Perhaps the same approach will eventually prove necessary for questions of personal morality and ways of living, especially when there is no longer a single moral centre. Hart has suggested that the alternative to enforced morality may not be permissiveness but *moral pluralism*, "involving divergent submoralities in relation to the same area of conduct."[19] Hart suggests further that if mutual tolerance was effected, then general submission to the essential "moral minimum" – Mill's rule of not allowing harm to any other individual – might be made more likely.

It is in this spirit of tolerance and moral pluralism that problems of drugs will best be treated. Already the young are evolving elaborate rituals surrounding the use of marijuana in the same way that any culture attempts to assimilate a dangerous but necessary means of altering consciousness. The problems posed by other drugs are by no means as straightforward or as harmless as those surrounding marijuana, but at least a spirit of moral pluralism offers far greater likelihood of solving such problems than the present spirit of narrow self-righteousness and vindictive repression.

Footnotes

[1]"Judge makes apology for jailing man, wife," *Globe and Mail* (Dec. 9, 1967).

[2]Alexis de Tocqueville, *Democracy in America*, 2 vols., (New York, Alfred A. Knopf, 1945).

[3]A. P. Herbert, *Misleading Cases in the Common Law*, 4th ed., (London, Methuen and Co., 1928), pp. 35-36.

[4]See Edwin M. Schur, *Crimes Without Victims: Deviant Behavior and Public Policy* (Englewood Cliffs, N.J., Prentice-Hall, 1965), for a full discussion of the concept of crimes without victims.

[5]Howard S. Becker, *Outsiders: Studies in the Sociology of Deviance* (New York, The Free Press of Glencoe, 1963).

[6]Joseph R. Gusfield, *Symbolic Crusade: Status Politics and the American Temperance Movement* (Urbana, Illinois, Illinois University Press, 1963), pp. 4-5.

[7]The RCMP has publicly stated that drug use is the number one crime problem in Canada today. "Drug Use top crime," *Ottawa Citizen* (March 20, 1968).

[8]See Richard Blum and Associates, *Utopiates: The Use and Users of LSD-25* (New York, Atherton Press, 1964), for an in-depth study of police attitudes toward drug users.

[9]For many of the ideas in these and preceding paragraphs I am indebted to Herbert Packer, *The Limits of the Criminal Sanction* (Stanford, California, Stanford University Press, 1968). See also the same author's review of the U.S. Presidential Commission on Law Enforcement, "Copping Out," *New York Review of Books*, vol. IX, no. 9 (Oct., 1967), pp. 17-20.

[10]Lord Devlin, perhaps the foremost contemporary defender of society's right to enforce standards of private morality, notes ". . . the simple and observable fact that in matters of morals the limits of tolerance shift. Laws, especially those which are based on morals, are less easily moved. It follows as another good working principle that in any new matter of morals the law should be slow to act. By the next generation the swell of the indignation may have abated and the law be left without the strong backing which it needs.

But it is then difficult to alter the law without giving the impression that moral judgement is being weakened." Patrick Devlin, *The Enforcement of Morals,* (Oxford, Oxford University Press, 1965), p. 18.

[11]John Stuart Mill, "On Liberty," in *Utilitarianism, Liberty, and Representative Government* (London, J. M. Dent and Sons, Everyman's Library, 1910), pp. 72-73.

[12]Devlin, *op. cit.,* pp. 13-14.

[13]*Ibid.,* p. 100.

[14]*Ibid.,* p. 17.

[15]H. L. A. Hart, *Law, Liberty, and Morality* (New York, Vintage Books, 1963), p. 75.

[16]*Ibid.,* p. 32.

[17]"800 Students Applaud police marijuana lecture," *Globe and Mail* (Oct. 27, 1967).

[18]George Steiner, "A Conversation with Claude Lévi-Strauss," *Encounter,* vol. XXVI, no. 4 (April, 1966), p. 36.

[19]H. L. A. Hart, "Social Solidarity and the Enforcement of Morality," *University of Chicago Law Review,* vol. 35, no. 1 (Autumn, 1967), p. 12.

Kicking the Habits

10

There are two habits we have to kick: the drug habit and the law habit. We would be much freer people if we could kick both habits 'cold turkey' and stay off them forever. Such an eventuality, however, is unlikely. But we could at least try cutting down the dosage.

1. *Kicking the drug habit.* "That humanity at large," Aldous Huxley wrote in a famous passage, "will ever be able to dispense with Artificial Paradises seems very unlikely. Most men and women lead lives at the worst so painful, at the best so monotonous, poor, and limited that the urge to escape, the longing to transcend themselves if only for a few moments, is and always has been one of the principal appetites of the soul."[1] And as William James said of alcohol: "it is part of the deeper mystery and tragedy of life that whiffs and gleams of something that we so immediately recognize as excellent should be vouchsafed to so many of us only in the fleeting earlier phases of what in its totality is so degrading a poisoning."[2]

The dangers of drug use are many. Any chemical introduced into the body with regularity may have deleterious consequences for the body, not to speak of the mind. Although alcohol and tobacco are 'acceptable,' their physical risks are well known. Amphetamines seem to be the worst of all the outlawed drugs in this regard; the practice of solvent-sniffing also exists way out in the never-never land of deliberate self-destruction. LSD is potentially very dangerous to the health and sanity of the self, but at the same time, it need not be destructive – in a sense this makes it one of the most dangerous drugs of all, for the very reason that the dangers are not always certain, and the risks are more attractive. With cannabis the risks would seem to be minimal, at least to a society willing to tolerate the ill effects of alcohol and tobacco. The opiates present a very difficult problem, for it does not seem that opiate use by itself causes long term physical debilitation. But prolonged opiate use does bring about a physiological change, after which the body will suffer if opiates are *withdrawn*. With most drugs, of course, there is a toxic dose level, and drug users are always subject to killing themselves, from the housewife taking an accidental overdose of barbiturates to the junkie taking an accidental overdose of heroin.

Addiction and habituation are the personal dangers most widely feared, but the more we find out about drug use the less we are able to say about which drugs are addictive, which create psychological dependency, and which are not habit-forming. It is extremely difficult to sort out physiological dependency from psychological dependency, and to relate these factors directly to particular drugs. More to the point perhaps, any chemical that acts upon the central nervous system in such a way as to alter the normal state of consciousness is capable of becoming an object of dependency. With heroin, tobacco, alcohol, and amphetamines, there would appear to be definite physiological signs of distress when the drug is withdrawn. But this does not mean that junkies, alcoholics, speed freaks and smokers are always in a worse position than, say, the heavy cannabis user. The physiological symptoms may heavily reinforce an existing psychological dependency, but even a dependency that is almost entirely psychological can be just as compelling. Peter Laurie points out that the sudden withdrawal of trousers will bring about in the average Western male many of the same symptoms demonstrated by the junkie when his heroin is withdrawn.[8]

A drug is taken to achieve a certain effect. If this effect is strongly enough desired, it will be sought again and again. The drug that helps one reach the desired state may eventually become an object of dependency. It is both as simple and as complex as that.

Dependency as such is not always harmful. Being dependent on persons is called *love;* being dependent on institutions is called *loyalty.* We all like to surround ourselves with familiar objects, whether furniture or pictures or books. Such dependencies are part of our identity, they help us to relate to our environment. There is no clear line separating this type of relationship from drug-taking. For example, when I wake up in the morning I drink a cup of coffee and read the morning newspaper. Caffeine is a 'drug'; a newspaper is not normally called a 'drug'. Yet both objects help me adjust to the situation of waking up. Coffee tells the body that waking functions must be activated; the newspaper serves to orient the mind in relation to the time and place. By continual repetition, coffee drinking and newspaper reading become the normal pattern of adaptation to the problem of waking. If one or both is withdrawn – if the coffee has been used up or the paper-boy forgets to come – definite withdrawal symptoms are experienced, that is, I become unhappy and short-tempered, and these feelings may color many subsequent actions throughout the day.

This leads to another danger of drug use, one that is not merely personal, but social in its implications. When drugs are used as a substitute for normal adaptive behavior, the individual becomes a less flexible organism. The more we lean on a particular drug to achieve a certain state, the less we are capable of reaching that state through non-chemical means. The more we use drugs to condition our responses the less we are capable of adapting ourselves to changes in the environment. The social implications of this point – and they extend far beyond the rather narrow range of phenomena examined in this book – is that the more we use drugs, the less adaptable mankind becomes as a species. One reason for the success that man has apparently enjoyed in the evolutionary process is the wide range of responses we have been able to make to changing conditions. Drug dependency is like a short-circuiting of the organism: its energies are directed into a closed circle. The more we use drugs to wake up, to sleep, to be happy, to be calmed, to be excited, to release inhibitions, to contemplate, to inhibit the appetite, to relieve pain, or the countless other actions we now use chemicals to bring about, the less are we capable, as a species, of responding effectively to the stimuli of the environment. A drugged individual is one whose behavioral options have been reduced.

There are specifically social dangers to excessive drug-taking. A drugged individual may be one whose normal functioning is impaired. We all know the hideous consequences of this fact for the safety of our highways, where it is quite probable that a majority of accidents are caused by drunken or drugged drivers. We speak of persons acting "under the influence of" a drug; such actions are not the voluntary products of the free will. A drugged individual is therefore a frightening spectacle to others: he is 'possessed' by a mysterious power; he may be dangerous; above all, his behavior is not *predictable* in the sense that most behavior is geared to other people's social expectations of how individuals should act. To others, the person, in a drugged state is an unknown quantity, an X. With familiarity this enigmatic quality may be reduced. Drunkenness is a common enough spectacle in our society that most of us are able to make quick adjustments when confronted with an inebriate. One of the reasons why people are so ferociously hostile to users of an unfamiliar drug is that they do not understand its effects. A tipsy gentleman at a street corner is a nuisance; a teen-ager stoned on pot is a menace. The *actual* effects may be quite different, but people are always most afraid of what they least understand.

Human beings are always trying to extend themselves. But the technological extension of human powers always has its bad side – in ultimate terms, we never get something for nothing. In Greek mythology, Daedalus, the great craftsman, designed wings with which he and his son Icarus could fly. But, intoxicated with his power to fly, Icarus went too high, too close to the sun. The wax that held the wings together melted and Icarus plunged to his death. The rampant technology of the twentieth century has given us the delusion that there is nothing that cannot be reduced to the level of a simple technical problem. And only now are we finally beginning to recognize the evil side of technology; its dehumanization of man and its poisoning of the environment. Drugs may seem to extend our capacities at any given moment, but never fear, the reckoning will come eventually, and accounts will have to be settled for the wilful pollution of the internal ecology of the person. It is a very old piece of human wisdom that the magical fulfilment of wishes always bears a price. The genie that arises from the magical lamp offers three wishes, but their enactment always ends in tragedy.

The use of any drug has a potential for personal and social danger. But living without drugs is a state that is only possible for a few persons. When Boswell saw a drunken gentleman, he asked Dr. Johnson why a man makes a beast of himself. Dr. Johnson replied that a man makes a beast of himself to forget the pain of being a man. So long as the human condition is one of pain and suffering, people will seek some means of escape. But it cannot be emphasized too often that drug use is much more a symptom than a cause of personal and social disorder. The real problems lie in the motives for drug use.

Public education is an essential ingredient of any attempt to cope with drug problems. But such education should not be directed specifically at youth and at the new or unfamiliar drugs youth employs. The drug culture is as much or more an adult phenomenon, and alcohol and tobacco are by far our major drug problems, even among youth. All drugs, whether acceptable or unacceptable by conventional standards, must be treated in exactly the same light. The affluent middle-aged pillhead with his Bennies and Dexies and sleeping pills is no more and no less a social problem than the teen-age pothead. Because the former is politically, economically, and socially powerful and the latter powerless ought to have nothing whatever to do with education about the dangers of drugs. If it does, then such an educational program will be quickly discredited as just another tool for the maintenance of the establishment. An educational program must also be free of puritanical or prohibitionist morality. Nothing will be served by refusing to recognize the lasting place of drug intoxication in human society. Finally, an educational program should not look at drugs in isolation, but must encompass the problems that give rise to drug use. Sound and unhysterical presentation of scientific information on the drugs themselves is necessary, but much more important is the attempt to deal with the underlying problems.

There are no glib answers to these problems; indeed there is not even much agreement on what the problems are. The special committee set up by Health Minister Munro is supposed to look into such matters. But all too often official inquiries either suggest a bit of minor fiddling with this or that detail, or else talk in airy terms about 'alienation', 'lack of communication', 'problems of human adjustment', or 'breakdown of traditional moral values' without ever relating these concepts to specific proposals for social change. My own view is that the soil from which drug problems sprout is not going to disappear until such time as the economic, social, and political substratum of our society of compulsive personal consumption undergoes some basic structural change and becomes reoriented toward community-centred rather than self-centred values. But that, as they say, is another story altogether. It would be amusing to see the reaction of those most concerned with the teen-age dope menace if they began to realize that the best way to take kids off drugs is to encourage them to join the revolution against the capitalist-bureaucratic system.

2. *Kicking the law habit.* The wise old anarchist philosopher, Prince Peter Kropotkin, said that "instead of themselves altering

what is bad, people begin by demanding a *law* to alter it".[4] Too many people have a touching faith in the magical power of actions undertaken by the State, or in the name of 'the Law'. It needs repeating that laws are made by human beings, enforced by human beings, and broken by human beings. Because one group of people calls itself the State, that does not, in itself, give that group the practical means of enforcing behavior patterns upon others. If enough people, in their wisdom or in their stupidity, decide to smoke pot, then all the rituals and incantations of parliamentary debate, the passage of laws, and the sentencing of offenders, will not change the motives of those who use the drug. If the demand exists, it will be serviced. Fifty years of anti-narcotics laws in this country have not rid us of heroin addicts.

The first delusion of lawmakers is to imagine that the law is a *thing* that can accomplish goals that people themselves are incapable of achieving. The law is only a particular form of relationship between *people*: if the people fail, the law fails along with them. The second delusion is to suppose that we can talk meaningfully about using the law to *eliminate* offending drug behavior. This is not only a delusion but a pernicious delusion, for it encourages precisely the kind of coercive extremism that has made our narcotics laws a nightmare of inefficient authoritarianism. "Just 5,000 more Marines, Mr. President, and we'll have the Viet Cong licked." "Add another ten years on to the penalties, and we'll have this dope menace licked."

The third, and most dangerous, delusion is that the law can be used to make people good. The law exists to protect people from others. We put people in prison because we are afraid of them. Despite all the rhetoric about "reform" and "rehabilitation," prisons are graduate schools for crime, where the first offender acquires the skills of the trade from the old professionals. If we were really interested in rehabilitation, would we treat a prison record as a lifetime stigma? Putting marijuana smokers in such a situation is a pathological misuse of power, especially when it is justified on the grounds that it 'helps' them.

Only occasionally are prison sentences for marijuana offences justified any more by the claim that the offender is being 'helped'. More often they are justified by reason of the 'protection' of the community. In the report that led to the passage of our first anti-narcotics law in 1908, a youthful MacKenzie King concluded with the following plea: "To be indifferent to the growth of such an evil in Canada would be inconsistent with those principles of morality which ought to govern the conduct of a Christian nation."[5] In the fifty years since, we have never really got beyond that statement. It is time we did.

The State is under no obligation to make it easy for people to harm themselves physically. It may even be suggested that an obligation does exist to actively discourage such activity. But two points must be emphasized. First, if it sets out to protect people from themselves, the State ought to make absolutely certain that its cure is not worse than the disease itself. Second, if it is not physical well-being that the State wishes to protect, but rather the 'moral fibre' of the individual, then such intervention is quite simply a totalitarian intrusion into the hearts and minds of people, where a democratic State has no right to be. As such it should be fought with the same indignation with which attacks on freedom of speech or of the press are fought.

In the case of protecting the health of its citizens, a certain amount of coercion may have to be exercised by the State. Drug-dependent persons are, by the very fact of their dependence, not entirely capable of exercising their own free will. But coercion untouched by any other considerations is bound to fail. Some attempt must be made to reach the person on a meaningful personal level. What we need is a more user-oriented philosophy of therapy. What we need a good deal less of, is the attitude described by Dr. Lionel Solursh of the University of Toronto, when hospitals and doctors often reject young drug users as "hippie dope addicts" even when they are in obvious need of of treatment. In one case a young speed addict went to four Toronto hospitals before being admitted for voluntary withdrawal. As Dr. Solursh comments: "Any doctor or any person has the right to reject human behavior but he does not have the right to reject the human being."[6] What we must purge ourselves of is the puritan notion that self-indulgence is essentially a moral fault and that its bad consequences are its own just punishment. Drug users need help, not moralism. Help will come when the drug user recognizes the self-destructiveness of his own behavior and begins to grapple with his *real*, as opposed to his merely *apparent*, problems. Too much coercion will not bring about inner assent to the judgments of society, and may only add to his feelings of persecution and helplessness and fix his attention even more firmly on the drug that offers him escape.

In brief, the medical profession must learn to treat drug problems not only with technical expertise but with the same sympathy and understanding extended to any sick person. To do such a job properly, an increase in financial support would no doubt be necessary to our already hard-pressed hospitals. If the government can afford to support vastly increased anti-drug activity on the part of police, it can also afford to help the hospitals.

The cornerstone of any overall policy on drugs will have to be a realistic response to the cannabis situation. At the very least cannabis should be removed from the *Narcotic Control Act* and sentences should be severely downgraded. Better than this would be the creation of a Cannabis Control Act, under which marijuana could be distributed by a government monopoly on the same basis as alcohol. The sale of the more potent and dangerous hashish from the East should not be permitted; many of the notorious problems of chronic cannabis use in the East are associated with hashish, but not with the milder equivalents of North American marijuana. Such a procedure would have the following benefits: it would merely rationalize an existing situation, which the law is powerless to change in any event; it would take the profits out of the hands of private entrepreneurs and organized criminal elements – where it is not even taxable – and into the public treasury; by separating marijuana from hashish it would allow us to at least partially uphold our international obligations on narcotic control; it would represent a flexible and liberal response to changing values of youth; it would greatly enhance the respect afforded to education on the dangers of more powerful drugs; there would be strict quality control and dosage uniformity; it would help draw young people away from the drug subculture that has provided the only source of marijuana up to now; in a stroke it would vastly relieve the jails, courts, and law enforcement agencies of one of their worst headaches. Persons now serving terms for marijuana offences should be released, and all records of such sentences should be expunged.

The proposals I have just outlined are sure to provoke violent opposition. Yet as Robert Fulford has pointed out:

Our society lives simultaneously on so many levels of opinion and experience that mutual understanding requires the most strenuous effort. In some circles the idea that marijuana should be legalized (or, more practically, that police and attorneys-general should simply stop prosecuting marijuana 'offenders' and let the law die quietly) is so old and well accepted that even to discuss it is hopelessly square. In other circles, at the other end of society, that same idea seems outrageous.[7]

It is my own impression that free use of marijuana would not change very much in our society. To an extent it may even be a more appropriate drug for social purposes than alcohol in a future of automation and leisure. Inasmuch as alcohol induces aggressive and belligerent behavior it may become less and less valuable in a society that puts diminishing stock in competitiveness and ambition. The point should not be overemphasized, however; both marijuana and alcohol can have different effects on different people. No doubt there will be potheads to deal with along with alcoholics, but the potheads will be with us even if the law does not change. Prohibition, after all, did not put a stop to alcoholism. But perhaps the greatest benefit of legalization would be a demystification of the cannabis cult. Expectations have a lot to do with the drug experience. Cannabis is forbidden fruit, which is usually taken to mean that it must be pretty damned good stuff. Books have been written in lyrical praise of the hemp weed, which not only make for dreary reading but appear ultimately to be much ado about very little. As one American writer commented:

If narcotics agents posing as hippies did not arrest children they put up to getting them pot, no one would be talking about marijuana, much less writing books about it. (Do Kent smokers read books about tobacco?) People would smoke pot as they have for centuries, but it would not be such a big deal.[8]

There is no equivalent case to be made out for the legal distribution of more powerful hallucinogenics. But steps should be taken to ensure that legitimate research is not inhibited, as now seems to be the case. Moreover, it is very doubtful that tough laws will have much impact on the use of synthetic hallucinogenics, because of the enormous problems of enforcement. Beyond this is the problem of natural hallucinogenics. Unless nutmeg is banned, all the peyote cactuses are uprooted, Morning Glories burned, Jimson weeds destroyed, and a host of other plants tracked down, there is no way that private citizens can be prevented from initiating drug-induced hallucinogenic experiences. The fact that the apparent link between LSD and chromosome breakage has caused an appreciable downturn in LSD use indicates that authoritative information may well be effective in communicating the dangers of such drugs, so long as the good faith of those dispensing such information is not open to question.

There should quite evidently be some form of tighter control over prescription of amphetamine and barbiturate drugs, since their misuse is a middle-class as well as a youth problem, and the source is more often than not medical. It is probable that both doctors and patients need to know more about how drug dependency can develop in apparently innocuous surroundings. More importantly from our point of view, some probing research needs to be done into amphetamine addiction among adolescents and the hippie subculture here in Canada. It may well be that speed represents a far greater menace to public health and safety than cannabis and LSD combined. But we know so little about it that it is quite impossible to devise an intelligent response without some factual grounding. A research matter of related interest would be to find out why so little public, police, and press concern has been directed toward the shocking effects of speed, while so much hysteria has been vented on cannabis and LSD.

Solvent sniffing represents a fairly clear-cut case of a drug whose harmful effects are beyond question, and are so baleful that stopping the drug use itself may be as important to the child's safety as helping him solve his deeper problems. Some combination of nausea-producing additives, age restrictions on sales, and an extensive educational campaign may help the problem. To use legal sanctions against children aged eight to twelve would be disastrous, as well as stupid. The whole glue-sniffing scene is one to give us all pause for thought: when kids this young feel so alienated and unhappy that they are willing to risk disease and death to seek an artificial means of escape, then what kind of a world are we building?

The opiates present the most intractable problem of all. It would be unfortunate if, in the current concern over youthful drug use, the heroin addict were to be forgotten, for the junkie, more than any other drug user, is a victim of the law as well as his own addiction. Concern over middle-class adolescents should not drown out the problems of the lower-class junkies. But here, more than anywhere else, there are no easy answers. We certainly need research; but this research must be undertaken without prejudgments as to withdrawal being the only acceptable solution: all possible approaches must be explored. We need above all to remove the legal barriers between the opiate addict and medical aid. It is possible for physicians to treat addicts under present law, although this would not seem to include the administration of maintenance doses.[9] A special committee appointed by the Canadian Medical Association to report on what constitutes good medical practice in the treatment of the narcotic addict found that "it may, in certain circumstances, be good medical practice to prescribe maintenance doses of narcotics for long periods to an addict at liberty, if other components of good medical care are also provided." They also concluded that "a cardinal principle of treating addiction is to focus on the patient as many helpful personal contacts and supportive influences as possible."[10] As for the law, its present distinction between the addict as a lawbreaker and as a sick person is very hopeful. It might be suggested, however, that treatment ought not to be confined to compulsory institutional centres, but that multiple approaches should be devised. Little quarrel can be found with long sentences against non-addicted peddlers and importers. It is a dirty way to make money, and when gangster importers like the celebrated Lucien Rivard are caught, little sympathy need be wasted on them. The addict in the street is a different story altogether.

One area of drug abuse that the law must deal with is the problem of dangerous behavior while in a drugged state. Such behavior can be in the form of aggressive or violent behavior positively directed at others or it can take the form of dangerous impairment of judgment, as with drunken driving. When the safety of others is endangered by drug use, then of course it is no longer a matter of the private morality of the user. But because A becomes a threat to others when using a certain drug does not necessarily mean that B will also become a threat when using the same drug. It is a very clumsy and inefficient means of protecting others to concentrate law enforcement on the drug rather than on the behavior that sometimes results from its use. It might be objected that prevention is better than a cure, but this really misses the point because, as we have been at pains to suggest throughout this book, behavior while under the influence of a drug is rarely, if ever, wholly caused by the drug, but is rather a product of the interaction of the effects of the drug, the expectations of the user, and the environment in which it is taken. Removing the drug from this equation may not be possible in practical terms, but even if it were, another drug might be substituted. It is the dangerous behavior itself that should be dealt with by the law.

There ought to be little objection to the ruthless removal from the roads of impaired drivers. Highways are an environment in which every move can have catastrophic effects on the lives of others. A report from Copenhagen indicates that Danish scientists have devised a urine test to determine cannabis use, although there has been no confirmation of this test by other workers in the field.[11] More research along these lines would be useful. It could be made a criminal offence to drive a motor vehicle while under the influence of cannabis, according to some objective scale. The law already includes "drug" as well as alcohol in the definition of impaired driving, and it may well be that many accidents are caused by drivers using amphetamines and barbiturates: unfortunately, we need to know far more about detecting such drug use. A good deal of research is required in this whole area, and perhaps a comprehensive piece of legislation with the emphasis on the removal of dangerous drivers from the roads rather than on *ex post facto* punishment.

Beyond this is the problem of temporary insanity pleas entered on behalf of persons charged with criminal offences committed while under the influence of a drug. In both Canada and the United States there have been a number of court cases in which pleas were entered that the defendants – on various charges ranging from theft to murder – were not responsible for their actions due to the influence of drugs, usually LSD, amphetamines, and glue (it is interesting that no such pleas appear to have been entered that named cannabis as the drug in question). The results of such pleas have been varied, but in some cases they were successful. In the United States, an insanity defence based on the use of LSD was accepted in a rather grisly New York murder case, as was a similar defence for a boy accused of rape and murder after sniffing glue. In Canada, the case of *R. v. MacIsaac*, which we quoted earlier in the chapter on LSD, which involved the defence of LSD influence in a series of robbery charges, was rejected on the basis that the voluntary consumption of a drug that alters the mind cannot be taken as the equivalent of insanity.[12]

It is to be hoped that the MacIsaac case will form a firm precedent for all other such cases. There is already enough confusion surrounding the use of insanity pleas in our courts; to extend this confusion to include a temporary insanity plea on the basis of a drug that was voluntarily consumed by the accused is to open up a veritable Pandora's Box of legal deceptions and loopholes. More importantly, if we wish to maintain the maximum degree of personal freedom in drug matters, it is absolutely necessary that we maintain the maximum degree of personal responsibility. *Anyone voluntarily submitting to a drug's effects must at the same time assume full responsibility for his behavior while under its influence.* The present legal situation is complex; the doctrine of *mens rea* – that criminal responsibility should involve to some extent a guilty mind – is a principle that would possibly modify the impact of the MacIsaac decision. But what I am advocating is not an interpretation of existing precedent, but rather a new principle that might be enacted in legislative form.

Another legal move that might be made would be to prohibit the *public* consumption of drugs, except in specifically designated areas. Tobacco smoking is a fire hazard and an imposition on the privacy of others when practiced publicly; marijuana smoking would be no less so. If more liberality is to be allowed in the private, voluntary use of drugs, then the obverse should be a greater sense of responsibility toward the rights of others.

The *Narcotic Control Act* and the *Food and Drugs Act* contain many provisions that are contrary to the idea of a free society. The burden of proof clauses, search and seizure provisions, and the use of special Writs of Assistance, are simply not justified by the gravity of the offence involved. We do not tolerate such procedures in murder cases, and it is difficult to understand how drug offences can be understood to be more menacing to the community than murder. All these provisions should be repealed. If there is to be respect for the law, the law must be respectable.

The community must pay a price for the weaknesses of individuals. Misuse of alcohol already costs us millions of dollars and an incalculable amount of human suffering each year. We are becoming more aware all the time of the costs of tobacco use. Misuse of other drugs – as much by respectable middle-class people as by rebellious youth – gives rise to extensive social costs, such as hospitalization and the waste of valuable human resources. But the problems do not start with the taking of a a drug; they go back much further than that. Moreover, attempts to stamp out drug abuse with outright suppression are not successful, and may well end by being more costly in almost every sense than the threat they are directed against.

Let us give the last word to William Burroughs, ex-addict and consumer of just about every mind-altering chemical or plant available. Burroughs was speaking about opiates, but his words are generally true: "What makes a cure stick is when the cured addict finds something better to do and realizes he could not do it on junk."[13] In a sane society there would be something better to do.

Footnotes

[1] Aldous Huxley, *The Doors of Perception* (Harmondsworth, Middlesex, Penguin Books, 1959), p. 51.

[2] William James, *The Varieties of Religious Experience: a Study in Human Nature* (New York, New American Library, new edition, 1958), p. 297.

[3] Peter Laurie, *Drugs: Medical, Psychological, and Social Facts* (Harmondsworth, Middlesex, Penguin Books, 1967), p. 14.

[4] Peter Kropotkin, "Law, the Supporter of Crime," in Leonard I. Krimerman and Lewis Perry, eds., *Patterns of Anarchy: a Collection of Writings in the Anarchist Tradition* (New York, Doubleday & Co., 1966), p. 289.

[5] William Lyon MacKenzie King, C.M.G. (Deputy Minister of Labour), *Report on the Need for the Suppression of the Opium Traffic in Canada* (Ottawa, Queen's Printer, 1908), p. 13.

[6] Joan Hollobon, "Psychiatrist tells of doctors rejecting drug users as 'hippie dope addicts'," *Globe and Mail* (Jan. 28, 1969).

[7] Robert Fulford in *Saturday Night* (May, 1969), p. 17.

[8] David Sanford, "Potpourri," *The New York Times Book Review* (Oct. 22, 1967), p. 18.

[9] R. St.J. Macdonald, "Narcotics, Addicts and the Law," *Addictions*, vol. XI, no. 1 (Summer, 1964), pp. 30-33.

[10] Dr. J. K. W. Ferguson *et al*, "Good Medical Practice in the Care of the Narcotic Addict" (A Report Prepared by a Special Committee Appointed by the Executive Committee of the Canadian Medical Association), *Addictions*, vol. XII, no. 2 (Fall, 1965), p. 37.

[11] "Researchers devise urine test that seeks out users of marijuana," *Globe and Mail* (Jan. 11, 1968). Some recent research in the United States suggests that under controlled experimental conditions marijuana intoxication causes less impairment of normal driving functions than does alcohol intoxication. In fact, the tests indicated surprisingly little impairment on the part of marijuana-intoxicated persons. See Alfred Crancer *et al*, "Comparison of the effects of marihuana and alcohol on simulated driving performances," *Science*, vol. 164, no. 3881 (May 16, 1969), pp. 851-54. It should be emphasized, however, that *any* degree of impairment is dangerous to other drivers, although it is perhaps possible that a marijuana-using public might be less accident prone than our present alcohol-using public.

[12] R. v. MacIsaac, Sudbury District Court (Nov. 8, 1968), reported in *The Criminal Law Quarterly*, vol. XI, no. 2 (Feb., 1969), pp. 234-40.

[13] William Burroughs, "Academy 23: a Deconditioning," *The Village Voice* (July 6, 1967), p. 21.

Index